A Caregiver's Guide to Lewy Body Dementia

A Caregiver's Guide to Lewy Body Dementia

Helen Buell Whitworth, MS, BSN

James Whitworth
Lewy Body Dementia Association Co-founder

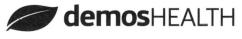 **demos**HEALTH

NEW YORK

Acquisitions Editor: Noreen Henson
Cover Design: Steve Pisano
Compositor: Absolute Service, Inc.
Printer: Hamilton Printing Company

Visit our website at www.demoshealth.com

Library of Congress Cataloging-in-Publication Data

Whitworth, Helen Buell.
  A caregiver's guide to Lewy body dementia / Helen Buell Whitworth, James Whitworth.
      p. cm.
  Includes bibliographical references and index.
  ISBN 978-1-932603-93-4 (alk. paper)
  1. Lewy body dementia—Popular works. I. Whitworth, James. II. Title.
  RC521.W45 2011
  616.8'3—dc22
                                2010038892

Special discounts on bulk quantities of Demos Health books are available to corporations, professional associations, pharmaceutical companies, health care organizations, and other qualifying groups. For details, please contact:

Special Sales Department
Demos Medical Publishing
11 W. 42nd Street
New York, NY 10036
Phone: 800-532-8663 or 212-683-0072
Fax: 212-941-7842
E-mail: rsantana@demosmedpub.com

Made in the United States of America

10 11 12 13   5 4 3 2 1

*This book is dedicated to our loved ones:
Anique, in whose memory Jim carries out
his mission of awareness
and Lucille, who was a dedicated teacher
and would be glad to know she is
still teaching.*

Contents

Introduction

In 1999, James (Jim) Whitworth's wife, Anique, was diagnosed with Alzheimer's disease (AD). However, when Jim looked up her symptoms on the Internet he found that they matched Lewy body dementia (LBD) better. "I told Anique's doctors about my research," Jim tells our audiences, "but none of them listened. They said things like 'Never heard of it!' and continued to treat her as though she had AD." We know now that some medications considered safe for AD patients can decrease the quality and length of an LBD patient's life. Jim believes that this happened with Anique. She reacted poorly to certain medications, her health went downhill quickly, and she died in 2003. After her death, Jim committed himself to increasing LBD awareness and support for LBD caregivers in the medical community and the public. With four other caregivers, he co-founded the Lewy Body Dementia Association (LBDA), which has grown into a strong nationwide organization.

Then, in 2005, Jim married me, a retired nurse and past family caregiver as well. I joined his crusade. With his help, I developed a series of LBD training programs for nurses and other health care professionals that we have presented in various statewide assisted living and dementia care centers.

Let's Write a Book!

One day, after a presentation to a group of nurses, I told Jim, "We have a book here, with all the information we've gathered and all the stories we've collected."

"No," he said. "We're retired. We don't need to take on any more projects."

Despite his reaction, I started putting everything together and, sure enough, soon we had a book. Before we go further, let me explain our writing process because it shows in the text. We have a partnership. Jim is the content specialist, and I am the writer. That's why when you read stories about us, mine are in the first person and Jim's are not. However, I assure you that this book could not have happened without Jim's enormous background of information, his ongoing exposure to caregivers, or his penchant for accuracy.

This is our second book. Because of my history as a nurse, and our training sessions directed toward care staff, our first book was for the people who help us care for our loved ones. Although there's definitely a need for such a book, we've come to realize that as much as paid caregivers need the information, it is the family caregiver and the families who hunger for it. And so this book is for you.

LBD families and caregivers have different issues than those who are paid to work with our loved ones. We know because Jim and I are both past caregivers—Jim of Anique and I of my sister, Lucille, whom you'll meet later.

Throughout this book you'll find personal experiences about living with LBD. Some are about real live people. Jim will be sharing some of his and Anique's experiences during their journey with LBD, and I'll share some of my own experiences with Lucille, who had Parkinson's disease. Some of our friends, such as Barbara Hutchinson, of *LBD Drive Across America*[1] fame, and John Young, past president of the LBDA, have agreed to share their experiences with their now-deceased mates.

Many of the stories are composites of typical LBD caregivers and their loved ones. We created the composites on the basis of several LBD online caregiver groups and forums that Jim continues to monitor and the many caregivers we have visited with across the nation through the years. I assure you that none of these people is based on only one person or family, although I suspect that many of you will see yourselves in their stories.

Because more men than women have LBD, we have chosen to occasionally talk about our loved ones with LBD with a generic "he"

---

[1] Helen Whitworth, "Travelers Extraordinaire," *Lewy Body Digest*, Spring 2007, 8, http://www.lbda.org/category/3477/the-lbda-newsletter.htm.

and about their caregivers, which are most often women, with a generic "she." This does not discount the many women with LBD—like Jim's Anique—or the many male caregivers like Jim. It simply makes for an easier read.

We hope you learn from our book. If you want to know even more about LBD, contact the LBDA or visit its Web site.[2]

Helen Whitworth

---

[2] http://www.lbda.org.

A Caregiver's Guide to Lewy Body Dementia

1

What Is Lewy Body Dementia?

So your loved one has Lewy body dementia (LBD)—or you have heard about it and wonder if that is what your loved one has. And if he does, what does that mean? How will life be from now on? What can you expect?

When Jim realized that his first wife, Anique, had LBD he had many questions, too. One of the first things he learned was that to understand LBD, he needed to know what dementia was in general. Then he had to know something about Alzheimer's disease (AD) and Parkinson's disease (PD) because LBD is often confused with the former and is actually related to the latter.

As a caregiver, family member, or just a good friend, you will want to learn these things and more. Do not expect the "experts"—your doctors, the staff at the residential facility, the nurses in the emergency room, and so forth—to know. LBD is such a "new" disease that they too are just learning. Our goal is to give you a head start in your journey toward a better understanding of this baffling disease.

Just What Is Dementia?

Isn't dementia just another word for Alzheimer's? What do you mean by "kinds" of dementia—isn't it all the same?
—*LBD class members*

Jim and I hear questions like this at nearly every class we teach about LBD. And I will have to admit that even though I had worked as a nurse in a nursing home at one time, I still did not really understand what dementia meant before Jim recruited me for his cause. Just like the people in our classes who ask those questions, I equated dementia with Alzheimer's. Also, somewhere in the back of my mind was this vision of a demented, irrational being. This inaccurate but common picture makes dementia a scary disease.

Although someone with dementia can certainly be irrational on occasion, the basic definition of dementia, which is caused by the death of brain cells, is much milder: "a lack of two or more cognitive (mental) abilities"—or, better yet, a *decrease* in cognitive abilities because, with LBD, these abilities are seldom completely gone.

Quick Definitions

- *Dementia:* A lack of—or serious decrease in—two or more cognitive abilities caused by the death of brain cells.

- *Cognitive abilities:* Mental functions or skills that we use to perceive, think, remember, communicate, and control our impulses. We often use two or more of these skills at the same time.

Dementia Is Not Always Alzheimer's Disease

It is easy to think that dementia and AD are always the same for a couple of reasons. First, more than half of the people with dementia *do* have AD. Secondly, dementias are seldom "pure"; they are usually a combination of two or more forms of dementia. For instance, Jim's wife Anique probably did have some AD mixed in with her LBD.

Of course, we have all heard of AD, but few have heard of LBD, the second most common kind of dementia. Vascular dementia is almost as common and better known, and then there are many other kinds that are comparatively rare.

> In her 70s, my mother had a series of tiny strokes. They didn't seem to affect her physically. She could still walk and talk, but with each stroke we saw her once-brilliant mind get a little foggier. And then she changed her diet, and her doctor changed her medication. She didn't have any more strokes, and her memory didn't get any worse.
>
> —*Mitchell*

Mitchell's mother had stroke-caused vascular dementia, which is not a degenerative dementia; that is, although each small stroke caused some damage, her mental abilities got no worse between the strokes. LBD and AD are both *degenerative,* meaning the progress of these diseases is relentlessly downward. Although there may be times when our loved ones appear to be better, such times will always be temporary. There is no known cure for any degenerative dementia, but a combination of physical, mental, and social activity, as well as certain medications, will slow the progression.

> The doctors said John had AD at first. Then they said he had PD. And then they changed his diagnosis to LBD. Why is it so hard to come up with the correct diagnosis the first time—and how can I be sure they have it right this time?
>
> —*Lydia*

Often, dementia will be initially diagnosed as AD. Then, as it progresses, the LBD symptoms may become more prominent and the diagnosis may change—or it may not, depending on the physicians involved, their knowledge of LBD, and the medications they prescribe. More important than the actual diagnosis is the recognition that your loved one has some LBD in his *dementia blend,* because certain medications that would be safe for someone with AD may not be safe for him.

> After my father died, the family had his brain autopsied to help researchers learn more about the disease. Daddy had been diagnosed with LBD for years, and it turns out the diagnosis was right—but he had AD as well. There were even signs of a few small strokes that we hadn't known about. That probably caused some of this dementia too.
>
> —*Andrea*

Families of people with LBD are encouraged to have their loved one's brain autopsied. This is one of the main ways that researchers can learn more about this disease. However, the arrangements must be made ahead of time if you want to participate.

- *Degenerative disease:* A disease that will become progressively worse over time. Although degenerative diseases cannot be cured, their progression can be slowed down. LBD and AD are both degenerative.

> • *Dementia blend:* A mixture of two or more kinds of
> dementia. Most dementias are blends with one kind
> predominating.

So Just What Is Lewy Body Dementia?

That is a question we hear often, and the answer can be a bit confusing. The basic explanation is that Lewy body dementia is an umbrella term for two related kinds of dementia: dementia with Lewy bodies (DLB) and Parkinson's disease with dementia (PDD).[1] Until 2006, when specialists agreed that the cognitive symptoms of DLB and PDD were essentially the same, the terms *Lewy body dementia* and *dementia with Lewy bodies* were used interchangeably. However, they are now recognized as separate diseases and, although some people continue to use a single term, the correct names are:

- **Lewy body dementia**, which describes both DLB and PDD;
- **Dementia with Lewy bodies**, which describes the kind that starts with mental symptoms; and
- **Parkinson's disease with dementia**, which describes the kind that starts with motor symptoms.

Over time, people with either type of Lewy body dementia will develop very similar cognitive, motor, physical, sleep, and behavioral symptoms, including hallucinations, insomnia, and acting out. LBD is a multisystem disease and may require a comprehensive treatment approach with a collaborative team of physicians from varying specialties.

Jim's first wife, Anique, had dementia with Lewy bodies. Because it starts with the mental problems one expects with Alzheimer's disease, dementia with Lewy bodies is often mistaken for AD, especially early on, yet the differences are there for the knowledgeable physician to see. Because of the serious medication sensitivities that someone with LBD may have, it is important that these differences be noted.

Our friend Bill had Parkinson's disease with dementia. He had movement problems for years before the dementia symptoms appeared. Although PDD is often considered just another symptom of advanced Parkinson's disease, it is in reality much more. PDD is a true dementia, with issues that often conflict with the movement issues of Parkinson's. These issues need the attention of a neurologist or other specialist trained in the treatment of dementia.

Biology

In all Lewy body disorders, tiny abnormal round structures called *Lewy bodies* develop in regions of the brain involved in thinking and/or movement.

> Lewy bodies were named after Dr. Fredrick Lewy, who discovered these tiny abnormal proteins in 1912 while researching Parkinson's disease.

No one knows yet what causes the formation of Lewy bodies, but we do know that *where* they form determines the symptoms we see. In turn, the symptoms determine what we call the disease (see Figure 1.1).

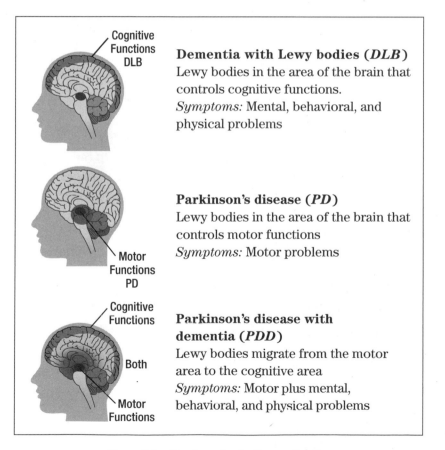

Cognitive Functions DLB

Dementia with Lewy bodies (*DLB*)
Lewy bodies in the area of the brain that controls cognitive functions.
Symptoms: Mental, behavioral, and physical problems

Parkinson's disease (*PD*)
Lewy bodies in the area of the brain that controls motor functions
Symptoms: Motor problems

Motor Functions PD

Cognitive Functions

Parkinson's disease with dementia (*PDD*)
Lewy bodies migrate from the motor area to the cognitive area
Symptoms: Motor plus mental, behavioral, and physical problems

Both

Motor Functions

Figure 1.1   The Lewy body disease family.

> - If the Lewy bodies are in the cognitive part of the brain, they cause mental problems, as in dementia with Lewy bodies.
>
> - If the Lewy bodies are in the movement part of the brain, they cause movement problems, as in Parkinson's disease.
>
> - If Lewy bodies are in both parts of the brain they cause both cognitive and movement problems, as in Parkinson's disease with dementia.

All Lewy body disorders, including PD, occur with a higher frequency in men than in women. The opposite is true of Alzheimer's, which affects a higher frequency of women.

Although uncommon, LBD does appear to run in some families. One of Jim's fellow cofounders of the Lewy Body Dementia Association (LBDA) had a grandmother, mother, and aunt with LBD symptoms. Naturally, her concern about this was the main reason she became involved in starting the organization.

Farmers and people who have lived in rural areas have a higher frequency of LBD. Therefore, some people believe that exposure to toxins, such as herbicides, can increase the likelihood of Lewy body diseases, but this has not been proved. Most experts believe that the cause is a combination of genetic and environmental factors.

The length of time from the first diagnosis to death varies from 2 to 20 years, depending on the general health of the person. However, it tends to be somewhere around 5 to 7 years. Death is seldom caused by the dementia itself, but instead by complications such as pneumonia.

Dementia With Lewy Bodies

DLB is one of the Lewy body dementias most often mistaken for Alzheimer's disease. Like AD, it affects the cognitive functions such as thinking and memory. Jim's wife, Anique, had DLB. Unlike someone with PDD, she had few movement problems until her dementia suddenly increased and her balance was affected. Symptoms not normally thought of as cognitive issues affected her sleep behavior and physical health and caused her to act out in irrational ways.

> *Dementia with Lewy bodies:* A dementia caused by Lewy bodies (abnormal proteins) in the area of the brain controlling cognition (the cerebral cortex).

Anique had problems with perception and sleep long before either she or Jim noticed any decrease in her memory or thinking abilities. She started having hallucinations when her dementia symptoms were barely noticeable. Later in her disease, she tended to faint when she got out of bed or stood up quickly. Finally, her condition worsened abruptly after surgery for an unrelated medical problem. All of these symptoms are common with DLB.

These noncognitive symptoms also apply to PDD, the other Lewy body dementia. They show up the same way, with some coming on before any obvious signs of mental impairment and others appearing as the dementia progresses.

The Parkinson's Connection

Parkinson's disease is also a Lewy body disorder, caused by Lewy bodies in the area of the brain that controls movement. My sister Lucille's PD symptoms included tremors, muscle stiffness and rigidity, slow movements, stooped posture, poor balance, and a shuffling gait—she needed a cane to maintain her balance. A schoolteacher who had taken care of herself all her life, one of the many things she had to have me do for her was to write her checks. She had lost dexterity in her hands and her handwriting had become so small it was hard to read. Both of these are common PD symptoms. However, she was still able to think, plan, and remember. Although I wrote the checks, she still told me what to write.

A masked face or blank stare is also a common PD symptom, but Lucille never lost the ability to show her expressions. Like Lucille, our loved ones with any Lewy body disorder seldom develop all of the symptoms that define that particular disease. Well more than half of all people with PD will, like our friend Bill, eventually develop PDD.[2]

> *Parkinson's disease with dementia:* A dementia that appears after a person has had PD for at least a year. The cause and symptoms are the same as those for DLB and PD together.

Parkinson's disease with dementia occurs when Lewy bodies migrate from the movement control areas to the part of the brain that controls cognition. They now cause the cognitive, sleep, autonomic nervous system, and psychological symptoms of dementia with Lewy bodies as well as the motor symptoms of PD. Thus, our friend Bill had both PD symptoms like Lucille's and DLB symptoms like Anique's. Besides his PD symptoms of tremors, poor balance, small handwriting, and the beginnings of a facial mask, Bill had delusions and hallucinations before his wife Barbara noticed actual mental lapses. He slept poorly, and Barbara ended up moving to a different bed to avoid being hit by Bill during his dreams. Like Anique, he had to be careful getting out of bed in the mornings to avoid getting dizzy and falling down.

Quick Facts

Lewy body dementia is:

- Different from Alzheimer's disease and related to Parkinson's disease

- Degenerative—not curable, but it can be slowed

- Caused by microscopic Lewy bodies in the cognitive and motor areas of the brain

- More common in men than women

- A disease that comprises two types of dementias that start with different symptoms but are very similar:

  ○ DLB, which starts with cognitive symptoms

  ○ PDD, which starts with motor symptoms

- A multifaceted disease with cognitive, physical, perceptual, behavioral, and motor symptoms

How Is Lewy Body Dementia Diagnosed?

It would be great if the doctor could just order a test and be able to tell right away whether a person has LBD. However, few neurological diseases, including Alzheimer's disease and all of the Lewy body disorders, have a specific test that can tell you "Yes, you have it," or "No, you don't." There is hope; some of the brain scans are getting close. However, for now, LBD is diagnosed using a group of symptoms called the *Lewy body dementia diagnostic criteria*. Therefore, the accuracy of a diagnosis will depend on how well your diagnosing physician understands the symptoms. Unlike in 1999, when Anique was diagnosed, it is now possible to find an LBD-knowledgeable neurologist in almost any part of our country.

If your loved ones' symptoms are among those considered closely related to LBD, doctors will diagnose their dementia as "probable LBD." If the symptoms are among those a little less closely related to LBD, they will call it "possible LBD." If the symptoms do not match very well at all, they will likely call it either AD or one of the other more rare dementias.

Because most dementias are a combination of more than one kind, a diagnosis of multiple dementias is probably accurate. For your loved one, the main issue is not the actual diagnosis but that any evidence of LBD in the mix be reported. With a diagnosis that mentions the possible presence of LBD, doctors can avoid dangerous drugs and provide better treatment.

Diagnostic Tests

Although the disease symptoms are the most important part of the diagnosis, doctors may use some tests to support their diagnosis. Methods that involve scanning the brain are becoming quite accurate, although the medical community still does not accept them as conclusive proof of a Lewy body disease. The two most common tests are position emission tomography (PET) and single photon emission computed tomography (SPECT) scans. However, live brain scans are usually available only in research and teaching centers.

The hope is that, eventually, the brain scans—or, even better, something less expensive and easier to do, like a blood test—will be available so that it will be easier to discover just what kind of dementia your loved one has.

Currently, the only conclusive test for LBD or AD is a brain autopsy. Although of great importance to researchers, they obviously are not useful in the diagnosis of a live person.

What Kind of Symptoms Does Lewy Body Dementia Have?

LBD is a complex disease. Besides the cognitive symptoms common to all dementias, LBD also causes other symptoms. There are medication sensitivities, which if ignored may cause your loved one serious harm: sleep disorders, one of which is so common that it is part of the diagnosing criteria; physical symptoms caused by the failure of the autonomic nervous system (the part of the brain that controls involuntary actions such as heartbeats); movement problems, especially with the kind of LBD that starts with Parkinson's disease; and, finally, psychological problems, or glitches in a person's perception of reality. If this sounds like a lot, it is; but it can be dealt with symptom by symptom. In fact, that is the way LBD is treated—symptom by symptom.

Formal Diagnostic Criteria for Lewy Body Dementia

DLB

Defining symptoms:
- Dementia (the central symptom; always required)

Three core symptoms:

- Fluctuating cognition
- Vivid visual hallucinations
- Motor dysfunctions (parkinsonism)

Three suggestive symptoms:

- REM sleep behavior disorder (RBD)
- Extreme sensitivity to some medications
- Abnormal brain scan

Probable DLB

- Dementia and two core symptoms
- Dementia and one core and one or more suggestive symptoms

Possible DLB

- Dementia and one core symptom
- Dementia and one or more suggestive symptoms

Symptoms that can support a diagnosis of LBD when they occur with core or suggestive symptoms:

- Repeated falls or fainting
- Hallucinations of sound, touch, smell, or taste
- Unexplained unresponsiveness
- Autonomic problems such as falling or fainting caused by low blood pressure upon rising, as well as constipation or unexplained sweating or coldness
- Urinary or sexual problems
- Delusions (false beliefs) or delusional misidentifications
- Anger, combativeness, sadness, or depression
- Difficulty swallowing, choking, or a weak voice

PDD

- Motor dysfunctions (Parkinson's disease) must have been present for at least a year
- Dementia (required)
- All other symptoms for DLB

2

How Do I Find a Specialist and Get a Diagnosis I Can Trust?

If you are reading this, someone you care about has probably already been diagnosed with Lewy body dementia (LBD), or you are beginning to wonder if he may have it. Let us start with the latter.

> My wife Marjorie forgets things—like how to do things she's done for years—but otherwise, we're doing fine. Although she and I agree that she might be having some early dementia symptoms, we're adapting and living with it just fine. Why should we bother to get a diagnosis?
>
> —*Carl*

Adapting is a great step. As with diabetes or Parkinson's disease (PD), someone like Carl's wife can have a productive life for years before the dementia becomes truly serious. Jim and Anique traveled extensively even after Anique had been diagnosed with Alzheimer's disease (AD) and had early signs of LBD. She might not have been able to travel alone, but with Jim along, they did well and had some very good times.

Making the Decision to Seek a Diagnosis

Carl and Marjorie also need to think about getting that diagnosis. There are two very important reasons for getting an early diagnosis. First, some dementia symptoms are reversible. Second, even if Marjorie's dementia is not reversible, a proper diagnosis increases her chances for the best medical treatment. An early diagnosis of even the possibility of LBD can serve to alert doctors to avoid prescribing drugs that are dangerous to people with LBD.

I'm concerned about the symptoms my husband, Dan, has been having. He's begun to drive erratically—not stopping at stop signs, for instance—and sometimes he acts funny and paranoid. And, well, he's forgetting stuff—like how to mow the lawn. I had to finish it up for him yesterday. He just kept mowing the same strip over and over. I want him to go see a doctor but I'm not sure how to get him to go without making him resistive. Should I set it up and call it a "routine physical?"

—Jackie

That might be one way of doing it, but, if possible, Jackie needs to get Dan's willing cooperation. If Dan realizes that his mowing is not right, or if he mentions anything about being forgetful, Jackie can respond with the suggestion that he see his doctor. That is what happened initially with Jim and Anique.

Anique told me she'd been forgetting things. That gave me the opening to suggest that she see her family doctor. She accepted my suggestion and went.

—Jim

Sometimes it can be more difficult. We tend not to mention mental losses because we do not want to embarrass or hurt our loved one's feelings—or admit to ourselves that this is happening. However, hiding from the facts will not change them.

Jackie is already concerned about Dan and has started to collect observations that show possible dementia. Reading this book or others on dementia, researching on the Internet, or both, can help her identify symptoms that may be significant. Jackie's next step is to share her observations and concerns with Dan in a nonthreatening way. It is best if he brings up the subject and then she can build on it. However, if he does not, she can say something like, "Honey, I've been noticing that you've been forgetting stuff, like when you mowed the lawn the other day, and I'm wondering if we should see a doctor about it. I've heard that sometimes, if you catch stuff like that early enough, you can stop it." (Yes, reversible dementias are rare, but it is a good selling point!)

Dan may be resistive to the idea, but he may surprise Jackie and actually be relieved. Alternatively, he may have been aware of his losses and too uncomfortable to say anything to her, feeling as if he had to hide them to protect her. Either way, Jackie needs to emphasize that it would be a good idea to see a physician and get a professional opinion. Jackie also needs to plan to go with Dan.

> When Anique came home from seeing the doctor she told me, "He said not to worry—it's just old age catching up with me." Then a few months later, I retired and we changed from a private physician to an HMO. When I went to collect our medical records to take them to our new doctor, the nurse asked me how Anique's Alzheimer's was doing. That's when I found out that she'd actually been diagnosed with dementia.
>
> *—Jim*

Although Anique had mentioned her forgetfulness, she was not willing to admit to dementia. Such avoidance is not unusual. Many people would rather not share, even with loved ones, that they have any sort of dementia. Jim's story highlights why it is important that you go to the doctor with your loved one. He made a common mistake when he let Anique go to the doctor alone.

Dementia is a disease the affects the whole family, so make it a point, if you possibly can, to accompany your loved one to the doctor. Not only will your support be needed, but you also have those concerns about odd behaviors and forgetfulness that you have been gathering in the back of your head. The doctor needs to hear these to make an informed diagnosis. You also need to know what to expect. If your loved one does have LBD, or any dementia for that matter, your life will change, and the more you know, the more you can plan for these changes.

The First Step: The Primary Physician

Usually, you and your loved one will see his primary physician who can then refer you to a specialist. Once you have made the appointment, start writing down symptoms and concerns as they come up, and take this list with you when you go to the doctor—that way you will not forget anything. If your primary physician believes dementia is at all possible, he should refer you to a specialist for a more accurate diagnosis.

> When Aaron started showing signs of dementia, we went to our family doctor. He agreed that my husband had dementia, but when I asked about seeing a specialist he told us, "No need for

that. It's just a waste of time and money. It really isn't important to know what kind because they're all treated the same. Besides, there are no totally accurate tests, so they'd only be guessing anyway." And he prescribed some medicine and sent us home. The medicine worked, and Aaron did get better, and we left it at that. Is the doctor right? Or should we still go see a specialist?

—Ethel

Statistically, more than half the people with dementia stay with their primary care physician and never see a specialist. A good share of these people will be diagnosed with Alzheimer's disease—or the doctor, like Aaron's, will say it really does not matter what you call it because they are all treated the same.

Years ago, when Aaron's doctor was in school, that was the case but it is not any more. Getting an accurate diagnosis is not a waste of time and money. We now know that dementia is a symptom of many diseases. Ethel, Aaron, and the physician need to know which disease they are dealing with because it could be one of the rare reversible or treatable dementias. Moreover, if Aaron has LBD, he is likely very sensitive to certain medications that are safe for people with AD.

Aaron's doctor makes a couple of points that need to be addressed:

- "All dementias are treated the same." This is partially true: The cognition drugs that work for Alzheimer's disease also work for LBD. However, this does not address the LBD issues of drug sensitivities, acting-out behaviors, or physical dysfunctions.

- "There are no totally accurate tests." This also is true; however you do not need accuracy. You just need to know if there is a possibility of LBD. Along with your loved one's symptoms, these tests give a good specialist the information he needs to make an informed diagnosis.

Choosing Your Specialist

In a best-case scenario, your family doctor has some knowledge of LBD, will want to refer you, and will know someone good to refer you to. Even if you are not so fortunate, your doctor will likely be willing to make a referral if you request it, and you may be able to request a certain specialist if you know of one. However, finding one can be the challenge.

First, let us talk about whom you should not choose. If your loved one has been exhibiting some of the behavioral symptoms of LBD, such as hallucinations or angry outbursts, your primary physician might suggest a psychiatrist. LBD caregivers view this as a very poor choice because psychiatrists tend to focus on the behavioral symptoms rather than the neurological issues that cause the behavior problems in LBD. They also tend to prescribe the very drugs that are most dangerous to someone with LBD.

If your loved one has PD, he may already have a neurologist specializing in movement disorders. Movement specialists often view dementia as just one more symptoms of Parkinson's and may not give it the necessary attention. If the specialist is focused only on improving movement, your loved one's cognition may suffer because the drugs that improve motor function actually decrease cognition. How the families of people with Parkinson's disease with dementia (PDD) must continually choose between mobility and cognition will be a theme that runs through this book. Someone with PDD needs a specialist who is knowledgeable about both movement and dementia, but as his condition advances, the dementia will become the most important issue.

As for the kind of specialist you should choose, a neurologist who specializes in dementia is often the first choice. Caregivers have also had good results with geriatricians, geriatric neurologists, and geriatric psychiatrists.

Kinds of Physicians and Specialists

- *Primary care physician:* A family doctor who knows a little about a lot of different illnesses but is seldom a specialist in any. He or she is usually the person who first diagnoses dementia, the doctor you will continue to see the most, and the doctor who will act as gatekeeper for the specialists.

- *Family practice physician:* A physician who specializes in general care of the whole family. (Usually another term for primary care physician.)

- *Neurologist:* A physician who specializes in diseases of the brain. Most neurologists have a further speciality such as movement neurologist, dementia neurologist, neonatal neurologist, or surgical neurologist. You want one who specializes in dementia.

- *Geriatrician:* A physician who specializes in geriatrics (diseases of the elderly).

- *Gerontologist:* A scientist who specializes in geriatrics. He or she is not usually a physician but may have a PhD.

- *Psychiatrist:* A physician who specializes in psychological disorders.

Recommended Specialists

- *Neurologist specializing in dementia:* These doctors are especially well suited to treating the LBD patient. Finding one specializing in movement in addition to dementia is good, too.

- *Geriatric neurologist:* A neurologist who specializes in the brain diseases of the elderly.

- *Geriatric psychiatrist:* A psychiatrist who specializes in psychological disorders of the elderly.

Proceed With Caution

- *Movement neurologist:* They tend to focus on movement over cognition, but occasionally you can find one who specializes in dementia.

- *General psychiatrist:* When unfamiliar with the disease, they may prescribe drugs that are unsafe for people with LBD.

- *Gerontologist:* Although skilled at working with aging patients, they may lack the necessary medical background.

How to Choose a Good Specialist

If you have a specific specialist in mind, such as someone whom other LBD caregivers have recommended, you can ask for a referral. If you do not know of anyone, start with your local universities and teaching hospitals. If there is a dementia clinic in your area, ask for the physician who works the most with LBD.

Most areas of the country have research and teaching centers. The Mayo Clinic has centers in Jacksonville, FL; Rochester, MN; and Phoenix, AZ. There are more than 30 Alzheimer's Disease centers throughout the country and most of them have people who also specialize in LBD. You can also ask at your local Center for Aging, the National Institute on Aging, or the local Alzheimer's Association about where you can find the nearest dementia clinic. Web sites for these organizations are listed in the References section at the end of the book.

You can also use your computer to ask other caregivers for advice. The Yahoo LBD Caregivers Support Group[1] has a caregiver-developed database of LBD-knowledgeable physicians and specialists. Although you must join the group to access the information, if you can use a computer at all, you should be participating in this group and in the Lewy Body Dementia Association (LBDA) forum. They offer a great deal of information and mutual support. If you do not have a computer, you can call or e-mail the LBDA helpline.[2]

> I e-mailed the LBDA helpline and got an answer right away. The lady said I was fortunate; there were a lot of LBD-savvy doctors on the list in my state. She sent me a list of all the specialists and I used a map to narrow it down to three neurologists with offices within 200 miles of our home. The first one I called wasn't taking new patients. Luckily, the second one was taking patients and I gave her name to our family doctor who agreed to refer us.
>
> *—Arlene*

Of course, you may not be able to choose your specialist. For instance, you may not be able to find someone recommended in your area, or your insurance may require you to use a certain doctor. However, with something this important you may want a second opinion. In some cases, your insurance may not pay for a second opinion, especially if you choose to go outside of their organization or geographical area, and you may have to foot the bill. Nevertheless, a second opinion is only as good as the specialist's knowledge, so it may be worth the extra cost to go to someone you trust.

Alex had been having dementia symptoms for over a year when we saw our first neurologist. We ended up seeing three different doctors who diagnosed Alex with three different things before we found one who knew anything about LBD. Finally, with this last one, we have a diagnosis that fits Alex's symptoms.

—Martha

Martha and Alex saw their primary doctor and the neurologist to whom she referred them. They did not feel comfortable with that diagnosis, so they asked for a second opinion and now feel they have a good fit.

Jim says he still finds many stories about families experiencing difficulties getting an accurate diagnosis—with devastating results when loved ones are given medications safe for someone with AD but unsafe for people with LBD.

My mother has Alzheimer's and Jerry's symptoms were so different from hers. I wasn't satisfied when our family physician told us Jerry had beginning AD. I knew it was more; his symptoms just didn't match Mom's or those I'd read about for AD. We asked for a second opinion. This neurologist asked questions the other one hadn't, questions about symptoms that Jerry had that neither of us had even connected with his dementia issues. I believed her when she diagnosed Jerry with LBD.

—Anita

Ideally, you will be able go to your appointment with enough information that you can easily judge the specialist's ability to diagnose your loved one. While we all know that "ideally" seldom happens, there are some things you can do during your visit that will help.

To check if your specialist is LBD savvy

- Ask the specialist the following:
  - How often he diagnoses someone with LBD.
  - How many people with LBD he sees.
- Listen to see if the specialist asks questions about the following:
  - LBD precursors such as active dreams, drug sensitivities, or motor problems.

- LBD-defining symptoms such as fluctuating cognition or visual hallucinations.
- Observe to see if the specialist includes you in the treatment process. Does the specialist
  - Listen to you and validate your concerns?
  - Ask for your observations and opinions?
  - Include you in the decision-making process?
  - Include things you can do in the treatment plan, such as behavior management, or does he focus only medical management? (You want a combination of both.)

If the specialist has worked with many people with LBD, and if he asks questions that show that he knows about LBD, you can feel safe in believing that the diagnosis is probably going to be right. If he treats you as part of your loved one's treatment team, you can feel comfortable that you have found a specialist who will work with you to make this unwanted journey that you and your loved one are on as smooth as possible.

It is vital that the physician sees you, the caregiver, as part of the team. Naturally, you want any doctor to pay attention to what you say, but when you are an LBD caregiver you are your loved one's advocate. Your loved one will eventually get to where he can no longer speak for himself, and you will become the expert on his preferences, reactions, and abilities. You are the doctor's eyes and ears. Because of the nature of the disease, you will probably see behaviors and problems at home that no doctor will ever see in the office. Many caregivers also find themselves being teachers to the specialists. Understandably, caregivers often have more time and incentive to learn about this particular disease than do busy doctors, no matter how good the doctors are in their specialty. With your input, the specialist can do a great job. Without it, the specialist is working blind. A Yahoo LBD group member put it this way:

It took climate scientists a long time to figure out that the Eskimos knew more about the Arctic than the scientists did and that the Eskimos could be invaluable research partners. It's the same with LBD caregivers.

If you do not feel comfortable with your first interview you may want to consider asking for another opinion.

> Jake and I had to go to three different neurologists before we found one who knew more about LBD than I did. The one we go to now is very good and we are so happy with her. I still feel as if sometimes we are paying her to use Jake as a guinea pig, but at least she listens to us and doesn't just brush us off.
>
> —*Norma*

Norma's story is not nearly as unusual as we would like to think it is. Lewy body dementia has not been a known disease for very long, like diabetes or Alzheimer's. It is so new that few doctors now in practice had a chance to study it while they were in training. Moreover, not all doctors, or even neurologists, and even those who call themselves dementia specialists, have researched or worked with LBD since they left school. Norma recognizes that, although Jake's specialist may not be as well trained about LBD as she would wish, they are better off with her than they would be with someone who will not listen and learn.

How to Choose a Good Primary Care Physician

Once your loved one has been diagnosed with LBD, the family doctor who referred you to the specialist will still be the physician you see the most. This doctor is every bit as important to your loved one's well-being as the specialist. He will be the one you go to for the many problems that come up in the life of a person with LBD and will often be the one to decide when you should see a specialist again. Therefore, you need to evaluate his ability to provide the care you want for your loved one just as carefully as you evaluate your specialists.

The family doctor needs to

- Have a basic understanding of LBD
- Know what his limits are and when to make a referral
- See you as a part of the treatment team

Good family doctors usually know the basics of many diseases and are skilled at knowing when to refer you to specialists. However, even more so than with the specialists, family doctors' openness to new information and willingness to see you as a part of the treatment team may be the most important requirements—even more important than their present knowledge about LBD. If your family physician fits this picture, you and your loved one will likely have good care.

Your Professional Team

LBD is a multifaceted disease that affects several different body systems. Before you are finished with this journey, you will find that the dementia specialist you choose and your family physician are just the start of the team you build to help you care for your loved one. Take the time now to choose the best ones you can, people with whom you can work and who are willing to see you as an active part of your loved one's health care team. If they are also familiar with LBD, so much the better. The time you take to make the best choices you can now will save you untold time and worry in the future.

3

Slowing the Progress of Dementia

I know that LBD isn't curable, but is there anything we can do to slow it down?

How can I help my loved one retain as much of who he is for as long as he can?

These questions are close to every heart of the caregivers of individuals with LBD. Moreover, as with cancer, there have been numerous ways suggested to "cure" dementia, or at least to slow it down. Most of the dietary supplements and herbal remedies do not work very well, if at all. Some drugs work even better for LBD than they do for Alzheimer's disease, but they are not a cure and, eventually, they become ineffective. The good news is that you and your loved one can make some lifestyle changes that, according to many experts, "work even better than medicine" to slow the progress of dementia.

Physical, Mental, and Social Stimulation

Although the use of vitamins and herbal supplements has not been very promising, we cannot emphasize enough how useful a regimen of physical, mental, and social stimulation can be. Although any one of the three is quite helpful alone, they work best when combined. The goal is to use exercise to oxygenate (feed) the brain and then use mental and social activities to "exercise" the brain. The old adage "Use it or lose it" applies to brain function as well as to the rest of one's body.

Exercise

Any exercise is better than none, but aerobic activity is best. Fifteen minutes twice a week is helpful; up to an hour a day is better.[1]

> David and I have been square dancers for a long time, and we still go. It's hard when he forgets some of the movements he's known for years, but we aren't quitting. This kind of exercise is just too important.
>
> —*Marie*

Dancing of any sort is great for our loved ones with mild dementia. It is aerobic, combines learning with sociability, and there is lots of repetition. And do not discount the togetherness, something that often becomes scarce for couples when dementia appears.

> Bill was an enthusiastic golfer until he became too unstable to walk alone. When we visited his family in Idaho, his brother and some buddies took him "golfing." They walked at Bill's speed, with Bill using his brother and friends for stability. Bill could hardly hit the ball but he loved being out on the course and being "one of the guys" again.
>
> —*Barbara*

Golfing is another activity that combines various exercises: physical, as Bill walks around the course; mental, when Bill tries to remember how to hit the ball; and social, when he experiences the camaraderie of male bonding.

Make exercise fun by choosing things the two of you like to do and doing them together. After all, your loved one is not the only one who needs to exercise. Walking, riding bicycles (consider a three-wheeler for your loved one), or swimming are a few other ideas for fun activities you can do together.

> The facility where my mom lives has chair exercises every morning, and I make sure Mom goes. She was very active until she became so unsteady that she had to use a walker. I think she is doing better physically and even mentally since she started exercising again. Mom sometimes gets confused when the leader throws in something new, but I notice that, over time, the exercises are actually all the same. The leader just does them in a different order to provide some variety.
>
> —*Marion, daughter of Clara*

Exercise should continue even after our loved ones are less mobile. Exercise is best if it is varied,[2] but for persons with dementia this can present a challenge. Sameness provides security for them. You can work around this by offering familiar exercises in a different order. Try walking around the same block but in a different direction occasionally. Or do one of two exercises on alternate days—walking on Mondays, Wednesdays, and Fridays with swimming on Tuesdays and Thursdays, for instance.

> Peter is mostly bedridden and seldom able to join in the chair exercises any more, but we still do exercises every morning. I get my exercise exercising him. We do them right in his bed, before he gets up in the morning. Sometimes, he can do a lot of them himself, and sometimes I'm doing most of the work, pushing his legs and arms around so they get some movement.
>
> —*Jenny*

Although it is best if Peter can move his own muscles (active exercise), passive exercise (having his muscles moved for him) is better than none. Even if you get some exercise working with your loved one, you should still plan more into your schedule, just for you. After just a few minutes of energizing activity, you will return to your caregiving job refreshed.

> The best exercise is one that includes physical exertion, mental stimulation, and socialization, lasts for at least 5 or 10 minutes at a time, and is fun to do.[3] Almost any kind of dancing, especially that done as a couple, will provide this.

Mental Activity and Socialization

Besides the mental challenges that come with exercise, quieter activities such as puzzles, writing, memory games, or working on a favorite hobby are all good mental stimulation.[4] I do not include reading here because it is just too easy for your loved ones to hide doing very little behind "reading." The goal is to keep your loved one active and engaged. How well he does the task is not important. His challenge eventually becomes that of maintaining a semblance of normalcy—of trying to remember how to do things once easily done and now quite difficult. Your positive attitude goes a long way. If you can focus more on the fun of the challenge than on the work, your loved ones will usually reflect this and become less discouraged. The activity must also change as the dementia advances. You want to challenge your loved ones to use their remaining skills, not defeat them with activities they can no longer perform.

> Mom started scrapbooking years ago. At first she had to make her scrapbooks "just so." Now when she tries to do them, she gets frustrated. But I've learned that we can have fun sitting together and reading her old scrapbooks, talking about the people and events in the pictures.
>
> *—Marion, daughter of Clara*

Clara used to make the scrapbooking itself her challenge. Now, that is too much for her. However, the books she has already done provide a vehicle for Marion to help Clara exercise her memory. Looking at them together is also a social time—something that happens less often as communication skills decrease.

> I asked my wife Janet, who used to love to cook, to help me put together some of her favorite recipes for our daughters. Unless she had the recipe in front of her, she couldn't remember amounts, but she could remember most of the ingredients. And she could remember things about the recipe—such as what she liked to cook with it, or even events that happened when she served it. I gave the recipes and stories to the girls for Christmas the year after their mother died.
>
> *—John*

John took a hobby that his wife could no longer do and helped her to pass it on to their children. Although it was a mental challenge for her to try to remember the recipes, the couple got to relive some good times together, and eventually their daughters received a very special gift.

When you can find an activity that helps your loved one to feel useful, whether it is a project like John's or just setting the table for dinner, you will find that it has a calming influence. That is because we usually feel more in control of our lives when we feel we are providing a useful service, and feeling in control is something for which persons with dementia fight a gradually losing battle. When they feel they are winning, even for a few moments, it has a soothing effect.

Here are some other suggestions:

- Ask loved ones about things in the past: family history, interesting times or events in your loved ones' life, what they did before they retired, or some special honor. Even better, get your loved ones to help you write about these times in their life, so you can share it with grandchildren, which makes the activity both useful and enjoyable. Consider recording your conversations if you are not comfortable writing them down.

- Get out a box of old photos and ask your loved one to help you identify them. This can be a time of reviving old memories for your loved one and can possibly provide you with new information. Again, it is not just a make-work project. There is a goal and your loved one gets to feel useful.

Socializing that accompanies exercise, as with Clara's chair exercises with other people and her scrapbooking with Marion, is not only very rewarding but also helps to keep dementia at bay. However, as the dementia progresses and reaching out becomes more difficult, isolation becomes easier than socialization. Eventually, conversation will likely become you and others talking while your loved ones listen. However, do not discount this. It is still socialization. Look for opportunities to visit with your loved ones, or for them to have others to visit with.

I always talk to Mom when I'm dressing her, or feeding her, or even putting her on the toilet. And not just, "This is what we are doing now," although, of course, I do that too. Mom doesn't talk much anymore, but I think she understands a lot of what I'm saying. I know she is less agitated [when I talk] than when I'm in a hurry and just try to get the job done.

—*Marion, daughter of Clara*

Marion is right on a couple of counts. Clara will respond better to everything if she is included—treated like the adult she is. In addition, the effort that Clara makes to understand what Marion says strengthens her mental abilities.

Diet

People who eat a diet high in fish, vegetables and fruits, and omega-6 fatty oils may have less dementia than people who eat other diets.[5]

Canola or sunflower oil, walnuts, and salmon are rich in omega-6. Although there is still no firm proof that these foods will prevent dementia or even slow it down, they are all good, healthy foods for anyone to eat. They are not harmful—and they might help.

Try to serve fish at least twice a week and offer vegetables a couple of times a day. Add apples, walnuts, pecans, or almonds to your salads, and then use a dressing made with canola, olive, or sunflower oil. Use fruits for desserts and raw veggies and fruits for snacks.

Just as with exercise and mental stimulation, eating a healthy diet is more helpful in a social atmosphere. Use each meal as a chance to interact with your loved one. Even when he gets to where he must be fed, you can still share and visit as you help him eat.

Dietary and Herbal Supplements

Several dietary and herbal supplements have been advertised as able to prevent or slow down the process of dementia, but none of them have a very good history of results. Worse, there are some possible dangers in using these nonprescription remedies, especially in the high doses sometimes suggested.

- *Coenzyme Q10:* This is an antioxidant that occurs naturally in the body and is needed for normal cell reactions. A study testing the effectiveness of coenzyme Q10 with dementia did show some effectiveness, although it was conducted on rats.[6] This drug has been shown to be safe in doses up to 300 mg per day. However, it is quite expensive and, to reach potential effectiveness, may require 1200 to 2400 mg per day.

- *Vitamin E:* Although this vitamin is a known antioxidant, it is oil based and cannot be passed out in the urine. Thus, if taken in doses higher than the recommended safe amount of 400 IU, it may cause damage. For awhile, neurologists pre-scribed vitamin E as an adjunct to dementia drugs, but because the amount needed is higher than recommended, they no longer follow this practice.[7]

- *Hormone therapy:* There are reports for and against hor-mone therapy. However, at this point, the danger of increased dementia (and breast cancer) for women probably outweighs the chance of positive results.

- *Ginkgo biloba:* You may have seen ginkgo biloba advertised
  as a memory aid, and it was once thought to be helpful, but
  actual clinical trials did not show it to be useful.[8] However, it
  is safe to use.

Although LBD is, in the end, progressive, you can use the preceding
techniques and ideas, and others you come up with on your own, to
slow down the process, to enjoy your loved ones longer, and to give
them some feeling of being in control of their lives.

4

Coping With Cognitive Symptoms

What Are Cognitive Symptoms, and What Kind Can I Expect With LBD?

Many of the cognitive symptoms of Lewy body dementia (LBD) are also common with Alzheimer's disease (AD), although they tend to occur in a different order. Others are much more common to LBD. Always remember that when we compare LBD and AD symptoms we are talking about what the dementias look like early on. The more advanced a dementia is—that is, the fewer live brain cells remain—the more it will have in common with all other dementias, although some differences will always remain.

Cognitive symptoms are caused by the decline of various cognitive abilities. These are the skills we use for perception, memory, thinking, communication, and impulse control. Usually we use two or more at once. For instance, as I type this sentence, I am:

- Remembering what I want to say (memory);
- Planning how I want the words, sentences, and paragraphs to appear on my page (thinking);
- Viewing the words I type as symbols with a certain meaning (perception);
- Communicating this meaning to you via writing (communication); and
- Staying at my job when I would like to go shopping because I know I can go later (impulse control).

Perception

We use our perception to interpret information from our senses: vision, hearing, touch, smell, and taste. For example, when we touch a piece of furniture, our perceptions tell us "soft" or "hard," "rough" or "smooth." A person with LBD, on the other hand, may not be able to tell the difference between a hard table with sharp corners and a soft sofa that will give when bumped into.

Likewise, when we hear a certain sound, our perceptions turn the noise into "bird song," but individuals with LBD could interpret it as a scream for help; they could hear the sound of a train in the distance as that of a nearby train about to run into their car.

> During one of our trips overseas, Anique saw a colorful scene on a TV monitor screen in the front of the plane and thought it was "fire." This was scary for her, but her dementia was still mild enough that she believed me when I explained what she was really seeing.
>
> —*Jim*

Anique was having illusions: seeing things that are actually present but seeing them differently than they really were. She saw color and light on the monitor and her perceptions turned it into "fire in the airplane."

> Anique kept bumping into tables and walls. We thought she needed new glasses so we went to the optometrist, who said her eyes were just fine. But she kept bumping into things so we went again, to a different doctor. This doctor couldn't find anything wrong with her eyesight either, but he ordered a new pair of glasses just to see if that would help. It didn't. Anique kept on stumbling—and complaining about her eye doctors.
>
> —*Jim*

Anique was experiencing problems with depth perception. Her eyes saw the tables and walls correctly, but her LBD-damaged mind was misinterpreting how close or far away they were.

We also use our perceptions to identify symbols. We perceive the printed words on this page not as little squiggles but as words and concepts. We perceive the sound of our friend's voice not as random noise but as identifiable words in our mutual language. As LBD progresses, it garbles these symbols and makes it difficult for your loved one to read or hear correctly.

Memory

Our memory is a storehouse. It is subdivided in many ways, but the division most important for LBD families to understand is that between short- and long-term memory. A functional memory depends on two things: proper storage and proper access to what has been stored. In a way, memory is like a book. Information is written down so it can be used later. If it is not written down, it will be lost. Once written, the book is put in a library, where it can be found and accessed over and over again, as long as it has been given a title, or "code." Likewise, the information in a person's short-term memory, that is, what is happening right now, must be "written" to long-term memory if it is to last beyond the present moment.

Like a book in a library, we find an old memory by the code we gave it when we originally stored the memory. If I attend a birthday party for an aunt, I might cross-reference this party in my memory as "birthday party" and "Aunt Jem" and even "fun" or "boring" as the case may be. When someone mentions Aunt Jem, I retrieve my memories about her party, as well as other items, like "skinny," "Ontario," and "loud," that I have also coded with her name.

People with Alzheimer's disease have difficulty storing information because AD blocks the gateway between their short- and long-term memories. Thus, what happens "now" does not get saved and is not there to be accessed later on.

> My grandma, Maude, who has AD, tells me great stories about when she was a girl, or even when I was little. But she keeps asking me the same question over and over.
>
> *—Janice*

Maude can remember what happened in her life before AD set in, but she does not remember Janice's answer to her question. The information cannot transfer from Maude's short term memory to her long term memory. Therefore, it disappears almost as soon as Janice quits talking, and Maude asks the question again. Because AD is the most common kind of dementia, this inability to store new memories for later is what we usually think of as memory loss.

People with Lewy body dementia, on the other hand, have more trouble retrieving information that has already been stored. Although the portal between the two types of memory (i.e., long term and short term) is not blocked, LBD causes a person's internal filing system to become disorganized. Accessing information from an LBD-damaged brain is like trying to find a letter in a pile of papers dumped on the floor and mixed around. The letter can be found, but it takes time. And if there are several related letters to find, they probably will not be found in the order they were filed. Of course, as the disease progresses, the "pile" gets bigger and the task gets more difficult and confusing.

> Anique gradually forgot how to brush her teeth. Sometimes she would try to brush them without using any toothpaste and then, when she was done, she'd squeeze out the paste onto her brush and look at it like, "What do I do now?" I had to start telling her how to brush her teeth, step by step. Eventually, I had to brush her teeth for her. Even so, Anique knew who I was and who her daughters were 'til the day she died.
>
> —*Jim*

LBD was garbling Anique's memory of how to brush her teeth—a task involving a series of steps that must be done in a certain order. Gradually, she lost her ability to access her memories properly until, finally, she could not remember how to brush her teeth at all. But she could remember the names of her family. Because remembering a loved one's name is not a memory that must be accessed in a certain order, someone with LBD will often be able to do this well into the disease and maybe even, like Anique, until the end.

People with LBD have problems remembering just the right word for what they want to say—the "I've got it on the tip of my tongue" syndrome that we all experience at times. And everything moves slower for our LBD loved ones, including retrieving memories.

> When I ask my mother a question, like what she had for breakfast, she takes so long to respond that I used to think she was ignoring me. Then she may say something like, "Breakfast?" (Long pause.) "Yes, I ate, uh, something." (Another long pause). "Can't remember."
>
> —*Marion, daughter of Clara*

Marion's mother remembered eating, but she could not remember what. The information was encoded, but she was retrieving only part of it. Besides processing slowly, she was having difficulty finding the right words. Clara has the kind of LBD that starts with motor dysfunctions, and her facial muscles are weak—a Parkinson's symptom—making it hard for her to say those words she *can* recall. Thus, her answers are long in coming and short in content.

> Memory losses usually accompany other losses, such as a decrease in thinking and communication skills and a general slowness of thought.

Thinking

We use thinking skills for planning, learning, reasoning, and doing sequential tasks. Sometimes these skills are called *executive abilities*. Executive abilities:

- Give our perceptions meaning,
- Allow us to be rational,
- Help us do more than one task at a time,
- Help us do a series of tasks,
- Let us plan ahead, and
- Allow us to learn new skills.

People with LBD tend to lose their thinking skills sooner than do people with AD. Many caregivers say that, looking back, they noticed a loss of executive abilities before they noticed any memory losses.

Hilda was a vice president in a large advertising firm when she started having trouble doing her paperwork. Tasks like completing routine reports became very confusing. I talked her into going to the doctor and eventually she was diagnosed with dementia with Lewy bodies. This allowed her to take an early retirement without penalty.

—Barney

Hilda was experiencing a loss of general thinking skills. Barney knew something was wrong and managed to get Hilda to go to doctor. Many times, neither the persons involved nor their family members will connect thinking losses with dementia. Thus, people have been fired for incompetence instead of being allowed to retire as Hilda was.

Anique was a first-class cook who specialized in French cuisine. For awhile, we had a business selling her crepes to vacationers at a local resort, so when I discovered a badly burned frying pan in the garbage, I was concerned. This just wasn't like Anique. But I respected her obvious need to hide her mistake and didn't say anything. Then a couple of months later, I retired and started eating at home much more than before—and I started getting regular servings of "burnt offerings." I quickly learned to cook! At first, I asked Anique for her favorite recipes and tried to make her a part of the cooking process, but soon I saw that she preferred not to be involved.

—Jim

Anique was losing her once-excellent cooking skills, which include the abilities like planning and remembering when to turn off the stove. Her apparent disinterest in Jim's cooking was, like the hidden frying pan, an effort to hide her growing disability. She accepted Jim's taking over the kitchen, her once jealously guarded domain, with grace—more evidence of her effort to hide her disability. Our loved ones are often aware that their skills are slipping, even if, like Anique, they try to hide it. However, not everyone is as willing to accept losses.

David has always been a methodical and careful driver, but now that's changed. A while back, he lost his temper because his car wouldn't start. He was trying to start it without holding the brake down. The next time he could start the car fine, but I was wishing he couldn't—his driving was becoming pretty scary. Finally, just last month, he ran a red light and hit a parked car. The state took his license away and his doctor won't sign for him to get it back. He's furious at his doctor! Although I understand how difficult it is for him to lose his license, secretly I'm glad. And I'm also glad that he is mad at the doctor instead of me!

—Marie

David's difficulty with starting the car was the same as Anique's when she began to have trouble remembering the steps for brushing her teeth. His LBD had diminished his ability to do a series of tasks in the right order—like putting the key in the lock, holding the brake down, turning the key on, and so forth. He missed a step, and the car would not start. LBD usually starts with short periods of diminished abilities surrounded by times when one can do the same tasks just fine. Therefore, it was not unusual that he could start the car the next time, although it does make it more difficult to see that there is actually a problem. A driver's license is such a symbol of adulthood and independence that David's angry reaction is very common—and understandable.

> About a year ago, Grandma Maude was still driving, even though she had AD. Then, one day she drove to the store and couldn't find her way back. The police brought her home after they found her sitting in her car in the middle of the road, crying. I came to visit the next day and while I was there I talked her into selling her car.
>
> —*Janice*

Maude was able to get the car started and drive but could not remember how to get home. Starting the car requires the use of skills already stored in the long-term memory, which a person with AD can access more easily than can a person with LBD.

> Before LBD, Grandpa Ed was a master woodworker. Then, we had to sell his electric saws and drills and most of his other stuff. He was still trying to use the tools although he really couldn't—most of the time he didn't even remember how to hold them. When he did get them to work, it was pretty scary— he wasn't careful with them at all. I was so sad. Grandpa Ed was sad too, until I dug out a box of old photos and asked him to tell me about them. Even when I'm not around, Mom says he looks at the photos and tries to figure out who is in them and what they were doing so he can tell me later—not that he can always remember, of course.
>
> —*Bernice, daughter of Kyla*

Ed had lost the ability to safely operate the tools he had used for many years. Even worse, he had lost the concept of cause and effect (the basis of safety rules), and so when occasionally he did remember how to use the tools it was not safe for him to do so.

Quick Facts

Memory skills:

- A barrier between the short- and long-term memories causes someone with AD to be unable to store present memories.
- A damaged "filing system" causes someone with LBD to be unable to find already-stored information.

Thinking skills:

- They are often lost before memory skills with LBD.
- They include planning, learning, reasoning, and doing sequential tasks.

Results:

- People with AD can still do old tasks or hobbies, but they cannot remember anything new.
- People with LBD have difficulty doing even old tasks, and their damaged thinking skills keep them from learning anything new.

Helping Your Loved One Quit an Unsafe Activity

When an activity such as driving becomes unsafe and must be stopped, it can be difficult for the whole family. Ideally, you should begin discussing the possible necessity early in the disease so that it does not come as a shock later. When the time comes, include your loved ones in the decision or help them to make the final decision, as Janice was able to do. Notice also that Janice—not her mother, who is the primary caregiver—was the one who talked Maude into selling her car. This decreases conflict between the two women who must deal with each other every day. If you know there will be strong resistance, as in David's case, then try to find someone outside the family to take on the role of "bad guy."

Hilda has always been so proud of her driving skills, but I could tell that she was making more and more mistakes. Way back when she was first diagnosed, we'd talked about how, eventually, she wouldn't be able to drive, and I brought it up again now. "I think the time has come, honey," I told her. "I think Lewy is messing with your driving." We have these discussions all the time about how Lewy is messing with her ability to reach for her cup some mornings, or making her forget stuff. And so it was easy for me to present it this way to her. She didn't like it but I noticed that she began asking me to drive her places. Just to be sure, I "lost" her keys to the car. I didn't want her taking chances.

—Barney

If early on you begin to make Lewy the culprit, not your loved one, and not anyone else, it is easier to talk about the problems—and even sometimes, to laugh about them. It also made Barney's job much easier than it often is for other caregivers.

Skill losses can be made more palatable for your loved one if you remove temptation as Barney did when he "lost" Hilda's keys. With Ed's tools sold and out of sight, he was no longer tempted to use them. It also helps to find alternative activities. People with LBD tend to be easily distracted, so you can divert them to a new activity, such as reviewing old photos like Bernice had done.

Emma was the typical farmer's wife, I guess. She had a huge garden. Every year, she loved the whole process: planting seeds, watching them grow, and then harvesting them. Even when we left the farm and moved to town, she had to have a big back yard for her garden. But now, she can't get around very well and the last time she picked up a hoe, she'd forgotten what to do with it. I built her a high planter that she can putter around in while standing or even sitting in her wheelchair. She can still enjoy growing things and when she can't figure out how to use the smaller—safer—hand tools, she uses her hands to dig in the dirt. Now, when Emma gets anxious, she goes out and works in her "garden." She comes back into the house dirty but much more content—and she even has fewer hallucinations.

—Howard

With a little work, Howard provided his wife with a safe and satisfying way to pursue a beloved activity. Such solutions are also often better than any medication for reducing anxiety; acting-out behaviors; or other LBD symptoms, such as hallucinations.

Assigning your loved ones a regular activity such as setting the table or folding the laundry is another way of helping them to practice the skills they still have. In addition, these tasks foster feelings of usefulness, which often have been diminished by their inability to do tasks such as driving. These assigned activities also provide structure and thus security.

Another thing that has decreased Emma's agitation is that I've asked her to do regular tasks—"to take some of the load off my shoulders." She folds the clothes when we do laundry and sets the table before every meal. Of course, she used to do all of this and more but gradually, I'd taken it over as it became too much for her to handle. It would still be easier for me to do it all, and I could certainly do it better. But her pleasure in being a part of the action again, and the way it calms her down, is worth all the bother.

—Howard

The following steps can help a loved one give up a loved but now-dangerous skill:

- Start the process by discussing the need for such a change early in the disease, so that when the time comes it will be an expected if unwelcome part of the disease.

- Align yourself with your loved ones against the disease, so it will be easier for them to accept that you are friend, not foe.

- If early discussion was not done or is not possible, get someone outside the immediate family, like a doctor, to impose the change—to be the "bad guy."

- Give your loved one lots of kudos for making a difficult decision.

- Do not leave temptation, such as your keys or tools, around in plain sight.

- Offer an alternative activity to fill the vacuum left by the loss.

Communication

Communication usually involves coordination between several cognitive skills and motor skills. We use hand–eye coordination when we write. We use hearing, symbol recognition, and verbal skills when we talk. Other communication skills are connected to memory, so that as we talk or write we call up just the right word or phrase. LBD affects not only the specific skills such as talking or memory but also the coordination between skills.

> I used to think that my dad didn't hear me but then I learned that if I waited long enough he'd usually answer. I have to listen more carefully too because his voice is getting weaker. And sometimes the words that come out of his mouth aren't the ones he means and I have to interpret. Like yesterday, he asked me for a turnip, but he was holding out his glass, so I knew he really wanted a drink. He knows it's the wrong word, but if we just laugh it off, he can accept it as part of his disease and move on.
>
> —*Kyla, Ed's daughter*

Ed takes a long time to answer because Lewy body dementia has slowed down his thinking processes. He must slowly process what Kyla says and what he wants to say in return, and even then he may still pull out the wrong word from his LBD-riddled memory. Remember that although there is usually little obvious muscle damage with dementia with Lewy bodies (DLB), facial and throat muscles will often be weaker, causing a weaker voice.

As communication slows and becomes difficult, the caregiver must look for other ways to maintain communication. This requires patience and intuition. Kyla developed patience when she learned to wait for her father's answer. Caregivers suggest that you silently count to 10 after you ask your loved ones a question. This gives them time to process and come up with an answer.

You also need to look for other cues to what a person with LBD-garbled speech means. Kyla used her intuition when she read her dad's nonverbal cues and guessed that he wanted a drink. Her positive attitude decreased his frustration and helped him accept his disabilities.

Successful communication also requires one to be aware of LBD-imposed limitations.

Several people in our family take turns staying with Aunt Callie, who has LBD. I go on Sundays, so I help her prepare for church. The first time I was there, I led her to her closet and asked her which dress she wanted to wear. She went blank and then started crying. We never did get to church that day!

—*Gretchen*

By giving Callie a choice, Gretchen was treating her as an adult and fostering feelings of self-esteem. But when Gretchen provided a whole closetful of dresses from which to choose, she overwhelmed Callie's thought-processing abilities and Callie became too stressed to function well. When a person with LBD is stressed, anxiety and some sort of acting-out behavior usually follow.

As LBD progresses, many of our loved ones quit talking almost completely. It simply gets to be too much effort.

Emma used to be quite a talker. I really miss that now. She seldom says much anymore. But don't get me wrong—she knows what's going on. I talk and she listens. When I tell her it's time to set the table, she does it. When I suggest something she doesn't want to do . . . well, then I admit that she doesn't seem to hear me.

—*Howard*

Lewy body dementia does not affect the senses—hearing, sight, and so forth—only the way they are perceived. Even though she has stopped talking much, Emma still hears what Howard is saying and comprehends well. (With LBD, comprehension is one of the last cognitive skills to go.) With this in mind, one should always be careful what you say around individuals with LBD. Their delusions can turn overheard conversations into something threatening. Then, because they are not communicating, you may not even know why they are upset.

Methods for decreasing the stress that can lead to acting-out behaviors, like Callie's crying, are addressed in Chapter 9.

Quick Tips

- Nonverbal cues are often more accurate than the spoken words.
- Delusional paranoia can turn overheard comments into frightening threats.

Impulse Control

Emotions are reactions to whatever we are thinking. We may feel sad, happy, angry, excited, optimistic, discouraged, impatient, or a multitude of other feelings. Although we often cannot control our feelings, healthy persons can choose to display the behavior they judge most acceptable for the time and place. This is one aspect of impulse control.[1]

I recently spent time with my grandchildren and watched them learning about these choices. Three-year-old Sarah ran though the house, shouting to her 10-year-old brother to chase her. Brian did not chase her because he had already learned what his mom was now telling his sister: "Sarah, stop running and use your inside voice. You don't live in a barn!" As we grow, we learn to choose when and how to show emotions like anger, affection, or excitement.

I watched Sarah struggle with another concept too. Brian could mow the neighbor's lawn and know that he would eventually earn enough money to buy the game he wanted. However, when Sarah did her chores, she wanted her rewards immediately. She did not yet understand the concept of delayed gratification, which allows us to wait for what we want.

Although loss of impulse control is not specific to Lewy body dementia, we notice it more with LBD because of the greater number of behavior issues involved. Loss of impulse control shows up as feelings expressed inappropriately, as the inability to resist unsafe or inappropriate behavior, and as the inability to delay gratification.

> Sometimes my dad starts demanding something to eat as early as an hour after he last ate. When I tell him he's going to have to wait, he doesn't seem to understand. He just keeps asking. I've found that I can usually distract him by giving him something else to do. I say something like, "Hey, dad, I think there's a good program on TV right now. Let's watch."
>
> —*Kyla, daughter of Ed*

Ed has lost his ability to delay gratification. Like Sarah, if he does not get something immediately, it is as if he were never going to get it. Kyla's distraction works because LBD shortens the attention span and makes it difficult to think about more than one thing at a time.

> David is only 50. He was a teacher who loved his work and got along great with his students. But a couple of years ago, he began thinking his students were laughing at him. I don't think

they were, but David was convinced. He used to be able to keep his cool even when the kids were way out of line. Not any-more. He started getting really angry and yelling right in class. Parents complained, and after several incidents the school superintendent said he had no choice except to ask him to resign. We'd been good friends with the superintendent, but after that he'd hardly talk to us. None of the other teachers would have anything to do with us either. It was like David was a pariah. When I finally convinced David to see a doctor, he was diagnosed with mild cognitive impairment.

—Marie

A mild cognitive impairment (MCI) is a very early form of either Alzheimer's disease or dementia with Lewy bodies, depending on whether there are memory (AD) or thinking (DLB) losses. In David's case, the losses were related to his thinking abilities. This early stage of DLB had impaired David's perceptions and his ability to make clear judgments. Then David's eroded impulse control was unable to keep him from acting out his hurt feelings with angry outbursts that fright-ened his students and angered their parents.

> LBD is not always a disease of the elderly. When a previously well-functioning person younger than 60 has no obvious motor problems but starts acting inappropriately, this may be the first sign of impending dementia with Lewy bodies.

Because of David's comparatively young age and the fact that his memory was still intact, his symptoms were misidentified by his coworkers and supervisor as inappropriate behavior over which he had control, rather than a medical disability. Because David had no diagnosis yet, he was required to resign to avoid being fired instead of being allowed to take a medical retirement.

Dealing with impulse control issues is often a matter of distraction and redirection. Fortunately, LBD also shortens the attention span, so if your loved ones want something "now" and it is not practical, do as Kyla did: Think of something else they like and mention that. Do not try to reason with a person who has lost the ability to reason. In Chapter 9, we suggest some management techniques that can be used to deal with the behaviors brought on by poor impulse control.

Impulse control is the ability to:

- Choose the behavior, time, and place to express our emotions;
- Delay gratification and thus build up resources; and
- Choose not to do (or say) something.

What Is Fluctuating Cognition?

Fluctuating cognition is common with LBD, but not with Alzheimer's disease, and thus it is one of the symptoms doctors use to identify LBD. Although Lewy body dementia is degenerative, persons with LBD may have times where they appear much better. However, these periods will not last, and over the space of months you will see a downward progression of cognitive abilities.

> Mom can be very confused one day or hour and almost as alert as she used to be the next. Some of the nursing aides in the dementia care center where she lives think she's faking to avoid participating in activities.
>
> —*Marion, daughter of Clara*

Clara is not faking. That is the way fluctuating cognition works. At first, a person will be quite normal, with occasional spells of odd behavior. Eventually, Clara's norm will become the confused behavior common to dementia with occasional spells of normalcy.

Quick Definition

Fluctuating cognition: A symptom specific to LBD in which a person shows various levels of awareness over a period of time.

> I go to see Grandma Maude about once a month. She has Alzheimer's and every time I go, she seems to be a little bit more confused. She thought I was my mom last time I visited, and this time, she didn't know me at all. I see other changes too. She's beginning to have trouble dressing and undressing and she doesn't seem to care what she says anymore.
>
> —*Janice*

Maude's cognitive abilities have declined gradually since the start of her disease. In contrast, Clara's cognitive abilities fluctuate from month to month, and even minute to minute, as her disease progresses. The chart in Figure 4.1 shows the decline of general cognitive functioning for Maude (with AD) and Clara (with LBD) over a 10-month period. Notice that although the cognitive functioning of both have declined an equal amount, there are differences: Maude's path is a gradual downward slide, and Clara's is more of a roller coaster ride.

Caregivers who spend every day with their loved one often have a different perspective than family members who visit periodically. Brian's grandpa, Harry, used to own a trucking firm that Brian now drives for. He visits whenever his route goes by his grandparent's house.

> My Harry seems to perk up when Brian comes to visit. And he'll sometimes have several days in a row where he acts so normal that it's like having my own dear Harry back, even when Brian isn't here. But it never lasts. With all his ups and downs, I have a hard time judging if he's had the general decline his doctor told me to expect. Well, except for his spell with severe colitis last fall. During that, he was really confused and I don't think he ever got as sharp as he'd been before.
>
> —*Nell*

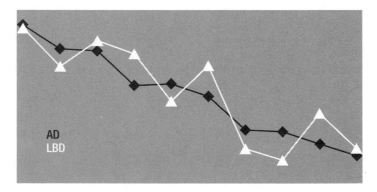

Figure 4.1 A simulated chart comparing the cognitive decline of a person with Alzheimer's and a person with LBD over a 10-month period.

Nell is there with her husband every day, and it is difficult for her to see the broad picture. Brian has a more global view of his grandfather's progress and can more easily see a developing pattern of decreased cognition.

> Grandma is right. Grandpa did get a lot more confused when he was so sick and he didn't recover all the way. But I think he's been declining all along too. He has times when he's quite aware, but they never last and the next time I see him, he's often just a little bit more confused than the last time.
>
> —*Brian*

The way Harry did not fully recover cognitively from his illness is another common story among caregivers. Such plunges will usually follow a "defining event"—a period of illness, an injury, or a drug reaction. Although a person's cognitive ability will usually improve, it seldom reaches the level that it was prior to the defining event.

> It was a very quick decline for Peter. He and I were doing just fine in the assisted living wing of this residential community before he fell. Peter had some mild dementia symptoms, but it didn't interfere with our active life. We traveled, had friends in for visits, and were foster grandparents. That all changed when he fell and broke his hip. He's not the same anymore.
>
> —*Jenny*

Peter and Jenny are both in their 80s. Even so, Peter was able to remain active until he went from mild to advanced LBD after his fall and the surgery for his broken hip. Then his awareness plunged and other LBD symptoms like hallucinations increased. He still had flashes of awareness, but they seldom lasted long and he almost never talked. Caregivers call these fluctuations *good times, bad times*, and *showtimes*.

Good Times

Good times are the norm at first, giving you an alert and aware person with periods of occasional confusion. The disease starts very gradually, with short little incidents of confusion and/or acting out. We just think our loved one acts a bit odd now and then, but most of the time he is as alert and aware as he always was, so we do not worry about it.

The occasional presence of these *good times* even after the dementia worsens is one of the big differences between AD and LBD. Maude, with AD, goes along in a gathering fog, gradually becoming less and less aware of their interactions with others. Harry, with LBD, has windows of awareness, during which he can relate with his family and has a better picture of what his life is like.

> Most of the time I had to help Anique brush her teeth, brush her hair, and dress. But sometimes, she could do it by herself.
>
> —*Jim*

Anique was experiencing a *good time* in which she was able to do the sequential tasks she was normally unable to do alone. As the dementia progresses, *good times* become less frequent and last shorter lengths of time. However, they never disappear entirely.

> Anique's dementia was so bad and she'd become so combative that I finally had to put her in a nursing home—something I'd promised her I'd never do. One evening, I was there in her room with our two daughters, Micheline and Jacqueline. Anique's eyes were closed and she hadn't shown any evidence that she was aware of us until Jacqueline said to her, "I'm leaving now. Give me a kiss." With her eyes closed, Anique puckered up her lips. Then Micheline and I each asked for a kiss, but for us Anique kept her lips firmly shut. Micheline had helped me get her mother into the nursing home; Jacqueline had been busy at home and hadn't been involved.
>
> — *Jim*

This is a sad memory for Jim because Anique passed away that night and that was his last communication with her. Although most of the time during her last days, Anique had not recognized Jim or the girls, she was able to identify them that night. Even with her eyes closed, she responded to each of them individually. Sadly, her poor thinking skills made it impossible for her to understand why her husband and daughter had not kept their promise to her, and she was not forgiving them. Even on her deathbed, Anique had a period of awareness. This does not happen with Alzheimer's disease.

Although this ability to become more aware, even if only momentarily, can be both positive and negative, caregivers tend to value these special times. A surviving LBD spouse wrote about some *good times* that showed up midway through her husband's illness:

An Old Flame

Yesterday I had a chance encounter
with an old flame.
He was every bit as charming as I remember,
and I was so glad to see him.
We had dinner together and talked
about everything and nothing at all.
It made me feel young again
and yes, I even flirted a little.
It was just so nice
to spend an evening being "normal."
I don't recall exactly when he left.
I just looked up and John was gone
and Lewy had returned.

—Lynn D., LBD caregiver

Bad Times

These are the times of confusion, acting out, and forgetfulness. As the dementia increases, the *bad times* will be more frequent and last longer until they become the norm.

> My wonderful, outgoing, people-loving Emma is gone most of the time now. In her place is this irrational, demanding, and overly possessive old woman. She wants to know where I am every minute of the day, and she's jealous of anyone who comes to visit.
>
> —*Howard*

Emma's LBD has progressed to where she has mostly *bad times*, where she feels unsafe unless Howard, her anchor to reality, is nearby and, preferably, focused only on her.

Emma will still have occasional periods of more awareness—*good times*—like Lynne's dinner date. However, this is a degenerative disease, and even when the *good times* do appear the level of function-ing will not be as high as it used to be.

Showtimes

Have you noticed that your loved one sometimes tends to appear more alert and perhaps even more physically able when others are around? Remember how Nell said Harry "perked up" when Brian came to visit? This is called *showtime. Showtime* is not something that a person with LBD chooses to have. Most of us have an ingrained impulse to show our best side to those we feel it is important to impress, such as the doctor and grown children. With *showtime* in effect, these people may see your loved one as much less impaired than you know he is. With-out impulse control, an LBD patient seldom chooses a behavior, it just happens. Therefore, you will not have much luck saying to your loved one, "Just relax and act like you're at home."

> *Showtime* has been a special challenge for me. Jake has become so combative that sometimes I can't handle him alone. I called Jake's son, Harold, and told him I felt that the family needed to consider moving Jake to a care facility where he'd be safer. Harold came out for a couple of days to see what I was talking about, and the whole time he was here, Jake was on *showtime*. Harold even suggested that maybe I had the problem!
>
> *—Norma*

Thanks to *showtime*, Harold saw his father acting much as he had the last time he was there. Jake was a bit absent minded, but he recognized Harold and was able to carry on a conversation. Harold knew his father had bad dreams and that sometimes he saw things that were not actually there, but he did not see this as a reason to place his father in an institution. Thus, he suspected his youngish stepmother of feeling tied down and wanting out.

Luckily, Harold went with Jake and Norma on their next visit to the doctor, a knowledgeable man who explained about the normal fluctua-tions that anyone with LBD experiences and about *showtime*. Jake was put on a waiting list for a room in a dementia care center.

Other couples have not been so fortunate. One caregiver's stepchil-dren went to court and had their father declared incompetent, took custody, and obtained a court order to keep their stepmother away. Because their father acted out only when he was alone with their stepmother, they believed she was causing the behavior.

It can also be a challenge for the physician when our loved ones act out at home but appear perfectly normal during office visits. LBD is treated symptom by symptom, and the best way for the physician to know what to prescribe is by observing the behavior causing the problem.

> Before Mom became wheelchair-bound and still lived with me, I'd have to take her to the doctor occasionally. As soon as we got to the doctor's office, she'd straighten up and walk better than she ever did at home, and then she'd slump again when we left. She talked better too—and her answers usually made sense. But it was really hard on Mom. She'd sleep most of the next day.
>
> —*Marion, daughter of Clara*

As you can see from Marion's example, it is not only the dementia that is affected by *showtime*. Clara, who has had Parkinson's disease (PD) for years, also had better motor skills for a short time. But *showtime* is very taxing, and it can take several days to recover.

Quick Facts

- *Good times:* The norm at first, these periods of greater awareness will become less frequent and shorter in duration but will never completely disappear.
- *Bad times:* Starting as isolated incidents, these times eventually become the norm.
- *Showtimes:* These are periods when a person involuntarily appears much more aware than usual.

Because you are around your loved ones more than anyone else is, you are much more apt to know when their *good times* are likely to occur. Use these times to your advantage—for sharing information, activities that demand a little more awareness, and times of special togetherness.

Mom is always most alert right after breakfast. She's rested and feeling good then. When she lived with me, that's when I'd try to get her to do some exercises, or work on her scrapbooking. Now that she's in a dementia care center, I've let the health aides know when these times are. They tell me it has made a difference in how much they can get Mom to do on her own.

—*Marion, daughter of Clara*

If your loved one is cared for by others, make sure they know when the *good times* are too. It makes their job easier and causes less stress for your loved one. You can also use these windows of awareness to share information or include your loved one in treatment or life decisions.

Peter is confused most of the time now. However, he still has short periods of awareness, and I've learned to save my questions and news for those times. For instance, when I decided to sell our car, I talked to him about it one morning when he was alert. Later, he didn't remember that we talked, but he didn't fuss when I sold the car and I had been afraid he would.

—*Jenny*

By taking advantage of Peter's *good times*, Jenny was able to provide a short time of normalcy for them both while they discussed selling the car. Caregivers report that their loved ones show less resistance to decisions discussed with them during these aware times.

A daily diary becomes an important tool for dealing with *showtime*. If you keep a record of your loved one's mood, behavior, and capabilities every day, you have something solid to show family and the physician. You can use your diary to support your concerns about your loved one's behavior, even when that behavior is not seen by others. The doctor will be able to get a much better picture of how your loved one's medication is working—or not working. Family members will also be able to see what daily life is really like. Of course, some people need more convincing than others.

A few months ago, I told our doctor about Jake's acting out, and I even brought in my daily diary. It just didn't seem to make an impression. And so, out of desperation, I dug out our camcorder and videoed Jake the next time he started trying to hit me. The doctor finally got it and changed his medications. After a day or so, Jake was back to his old self.

—*Norma*

Be creative. Norma's solution of using a camera worked for her. Perhaps all you might need is an audio recorder. Use whatever works.

How Are Cognitive Symptoms Treated?

No degenerative dementias, including Lewy body dementia, can be cured with medication. However, some drugs can slow the progress. These medications may make it possible for you to keep your loved one at home a few years longer before you need to consider residential care. Remember that physical, mental, and social activity combined with a good diet also slows the progress of most dementias.

Dementia drugs will reduce cognitive symptoms such as forgetfulness, confusion, and poor thinking abilities, along with other LBD symptoms. The downside is that the effects will not last. As more and more brain cells die, these drugs become less and less effective.

Three drugs, donepezil (Aricept), galantamine (Razadyne), and rivastigmine (Exelon), are all approved by the Food and Drug Administration (FDA) to treat mild to moderate AD but, with one exception, not LBD. The exception is Exelon, which is now approved for Parkinson's disease dementia (PDD). Nevertheless, there is a lot of research that show that these drugs may all work better for LBD (DLB as well as PDD) than they do for AD. These drugs must be used one at a time because their site of action in live brain cells is the same: They all work to preserve the amount of acetylcholine, an important chemical in the brain that is vital to concentration, memory formation, and muscle movement and control. Using more than one of these medications at a time can greatly increase side effects without increasing effectiveness. Dementia drugs do not keep brain cells from dying—they simply boost the action of living cells. As the disease kills more cells, the drugs become less effective.

When should my loved one start using dementia drugs? I've heard that they only last for a few years and then they don't work anymore. Shouldn't we wait then, until he really needs them so that they'll still work when he gets really bad?

—*Annette*

Your loved one can start using the drugs as soon there are symptoms to treat. The drugs do not stop working because of the time they have been used; they stop working because there are fewer live brain cells for them to act on. Using the dementia drugs does not make the brain cells die.

What Side Effects Can I Expect?

Possible side effects for all of these drugs include severe gastrointestinal tract (GI) symptoms such as nausea, diarrhea, and cramps. Exelon now comes in a patch that, because it bypasses the GI tract, decreases the GI symptoms. Dementia drugs also may cause or increase motor dysfunctions, a problem we cover in the next chapter.

> The doctor put Hilda on Exelon right off, saying that was usually the best drug for LBD patients. But it made Hilda sick to her stomach, so then he put her on Aricept, and that's what she's been taking since. It does help, and as long as she takes it with food, she has almost no nausea. Hilda is almost normal now. But I hear that the new Exelon patch has even fewer side effects, so we are going to ask about it next time we see the doctor.
>
> —*Barney*

Exelon does have the best track record for LBD and is now approved by the FDA for PDD. However, of the three acetylcholine-preserving drugs, it is the one that causes the most GI problems when taken orally. The patch, which bypasses the GI tract, may work better. Note that Barney is doing a good job of being an advocate for his wife. He is not planning to wait for the doctor to suggest the patch. As caregivers, we need to be aware of advances in LBD treatment, like the patch, that can help our loved ones and bring them to the attention of their doctors. That is often the way busy doctors with large practices and little time for research learn about them. A good doctor is willing to listen and check your information out.

Dementia drugs are all extremely expensive. Their average cost is more than $500 per month. We hope that will change, or at least that the costs will decrease as generic versions enter the market. Galantamine, a generic form of Razadyne, became available in early 2009 and donepezil, a generic form of Aricept, was approved by the FDA in early 2010 and will soon be available. Although generic versions are less expensive than the brand name drugs, "less expensive" is still subjective; monthly costs can still be well over $200 per month.

Memantine (Namenda) is the only dementia drug approved by the FDA for moderate to severe AD. Like the preceding drugs, it is not yet approved for LBD. Namenda works to preserve the amount of the chemical glutamate in the brain. Because it works with a different chemical than the other three drugs do, it can be used in conjunction with them. Usually Namenda is added to boost effectiveness when the other drugs begin to fail. Occasionally, someone may do better with just Namenda, but that is unusual with LBD.

> My husband, Peter, still uses Aricept. He's never had any trou-
> ble with it, and up to the last month or so, we've been happy
> with it. But I think it's not working as well anymore. Peter is
> having more hallucinations again. I just hope he doesn't get
> delusional again.
>
> —*Jenny*

Peter was responsive to the medication at first, but his dementia is becoming more advanced. The reoccurrence of hallucinations is a sign that Peter's present medication is beginning to fail. His doctor may add Namenda, which should help Peter's Aricept work better without adding any serious side effects, the next time Peter sees him. However, eventually even this may not work. All dementia drugs become less effective with the progression of the disease.

> Jake's been through them all. For awhile, we wondered if his
> doctor really knew what she was doing or if she was just playing
> Russian roulette and hoping something would work. But Jake's
> doing well on Razadyne now, and we are excited that they've
> come out with a generic. It's going to cut our drug bill down a
> lot! Much of Jake's drug costs come out of our own budget. Now
> it they'd only have generics of all the other drugs Jake's on.
>
> —*Norma*

Jake's doctor had been trying out different drugs to find the best fit for him. Each person reacts to dementia drugs differently, and the only way to tell which is best is to try them out one by one. Unless your doctor treats a lot of people with LBD, Aricept will often be the first one he or she will prescribe. Aricept has been around a long time, and doctors prefer to use the drug they know best if it will work. Do not discount this. Knowing a drug and its side effects is important for good drug management.

Dementia Drugs

- *Donepezil (Aricept):* Marketed by Pfizer and approved by the FDA for AD in 1996, this drug is not yet approved for any LBD. However, clinical trials have shown it to be possibly more effective with LBD than AD. The oldest of three acetylcholine-preserving drugs, Aricept is often the first drug chosen by neurologists. In December of 2009, the FDA approved a generic version.[2]

- *Rivastigmine (Exelon):* Marketed by Novartis and approved for AD in 2000, this acetylcholine-preserving drug was approved for PDD in 2006. Research has shown that Exelon may be the best drug to work with DLB as well.[3,4] In 2008, Novartis came out with an Exelon patch,[5] which greatly decreased the GI side effects that sometimes made this drug difficult to use.

- *Galantamine (Razadyne):* Marketed by Janssen Pharmaceuticals, this acetylcholine-preserving drug was approved for AD in 2001. Razadyne is a natural (i.e., non-manufactured) drug obtained from daffodil bulbs and thus, may have fewer side effects. In August of 2008 the generic was approved by the FDA, making it the first cognition drug to be available in this less expensive form.[6]

- *Memantine (Namenda):* Marketed by Forest Laboratories, Namenda was approved for moderate to severe AD in 2005. This drug's action is different from the preceding drugs, and therefore it can be used in combination with them. The good news for LBD families is that recent studies are showing that Namenda increases the effectiveness of other dementia drugs for persons with DLB and PDD.[7] This may eventually get Namenda approved by the FDA for Lewy body dementias.

The caregiving issues with dementia medications include the trial and error needed to find the "perfect fit" for each person, the side effects that each drug may have, and the costs. This is a team effort, with the goal of providing your loved ones with the best possible combination of drugs, or "drug cocktail," for their particular symptoms. Your doctor's job is to evaluate; then prescribe; and, upon learning of the results, refine the prescription. Your job is to be a good observer, record keeper, and reporter.

Look for possible side effects. If they are serious, you will want to report them at once. Often they will be minor and will not mean much by themselves. Keep a record of these and report them at the next doctor's visit. Every little bit of information you can bring will help the doctor attain your mutual goal. Remember, these drugs work on live cells. As more cells die, they become less effective, making this is an unending job. Even when you find the perfect "cocktail," it will eventually need adjusting.

Although all of these drugs have GI side effects; sometimes they can be decreased when taken with food. Even then, some people cannot tolerate a certain drug, and the doctor will have to try a different one. The motor side effects are more difficult to control. Again, the doctor will try different drugs, or combinations of drugs, but eventually the family may have to make choices between mobility and cognition. This is discussed at greater length in the next chapter. If cost is an issue for you, you might want to ask the doctor if your loved one can try a dementia drug that is sold in a generic form.

It is important to remember that all of the differences between LBD and AD discussed in this chapter become less apparent as the disease progresses. As more cognitive abilities become affected, the dementias will appear more similar. However, by then other symptoms specific to LBD, such as hallucinations, may be apparent.

5

Coping With Motor Dysfunctions

In the Lewy body disorders, movement problems are as big an issue as dementia. Most people with Lewy body dementia (LBD) will have some sort of motor dysfunction, even if they did not start out with Parkinson's disease (PD). Cases in which the motor dysfunction begins after dementia are called *parkinsonism.* A person with LBD may have any or all of the following symptoms:

- *Muscle stiffness or rigidity:* Muscles may ache or tire easily. This symptom is always present with Parkinson's disease with dementia (PDD). For someone with dementia with Lewy bodies (DLB), it is one of the most common side effects of some medications.

- *Slow movements:* Lewy body dementia makes everything slower—thinking, talking, moving one's muscles, and so on.

- *Muscle weakness:* Just as LBD makes everything slower, it also makes muscles weaker. This symptom is always present with PDD. For someone with DLB, this may be noticed most in the muscles that control chewing and swallowing.

- *Stooped posture, shuffling gait, and balance problems:* Problems with back and leg muscles may cause more balance problems for a person with Parkinson's disease with dementia than for someone with DLB. They can be manifested in someone with dementia with Lewy bodies as side effects of some medications. Low blood pressure upon rising can cause dizziness and loss of balance for anyone with LBD.

- *Tremor:* This is often the first sign of Parkinson's disease. It is most common when the muscles are at rest. In someone with dementia with Lewy bodies, it can be a side effect of some medications.

- *Loss of dexterity:* This is most common with Parkinson's disease with dementia, but as DLB advances dexterity will likely decrease too. Dexterity may also be affected by poor hand–eye coordination.

- *Blank facial expression:* Although most common with PDD, this may be present with DLB as well.

- *Small handwriting:* This is most common with PDD, but it may develop in late stage DLB or be caused by the side effects of some medications.

Motor Dysfunctions That Start Before Dementia

Motor dysfunctions that begin prior to the dementia are most likely caused by Lewy bodies in the movement control areas of brain, or Parkinson's disease. When dementia appears in someone who already has PD, this is diagnosed as Parkinson's disease with dementia.

> Bill had PD long before he developed any dementia symptoms. He took the PD drug Sinemet for several years, and all he had was a slight tremor. Then he began to have more problems— shuffling when he walked and leaning so far forward that he had to use a cane. But his mind was fine. In fact, he was still working as a carpentry teacher at the community college.
>
> —*Barbara*

Bill's motor symptoms were a part of his Lewy body disorder right from the beginning. Parkinson's disease, like all Lewy body disorders, is a progressive disease and so his symptoms gradually increased even though he was taking medication to control them.

More than just the muscles in the arms and legs are affected. Many people with Parkinson's disease develop facial masks. Their cheek and other facial muscles become so weak that they do not move easily, and their faces become expressionless masks. The weak facial muscles also make it more difficult to form words, which affects communication. Weak throat muscles cause the voice to become soft, and this, too, decreases a person's ability to communicate verbally.

These muscle problems continue to get worse even after dementia sets in. Masklike faces and weak voices are common in the more advanced cases of DLB in which there has been very little obvious muscle damage.

> Motor dysfunctions such as muscle stiffness, rigidity, or weakness; slow movements; stooped posture; shuffling gait; balance problems; tremors; loss of dexterity; blank facial expression; and small handwriting can all be present with Parkinson's disease or PDD and many may also be present with DLB.

Treating Parkinson's Disease

Drugs used to treat Parkinson's disease act to preserve the chemical dopamine, which helps the brain control motor movements. Bill's drug, carbidopa/levodopa (Sinemet), is one of the most commonly used because it is the most effective and has the fewest short-term side effects. However, it is associated with high risks of long-term side effects, such as rigidity. Changes in the amount or timing will usually prevent side effects, but experts now recommend that newer drugs, such as ropinirole (Requip) or pramipexole (Mirapex) be used as a first choice and that Sinemet be used only when these drugs fail to provide sufficient relief.[1]

Although Requip and Mirapex are reported to be better tolerated and do not carry the same risks of long-term complications, they have a much higher risk of short-term side effects, such as confusion and hallucinations. Therefore, they are a poor choice for anyone who has dementia. In addition, they have addictive properties and cannot be stopped abruptly because they can cause severe withdrawal symptoms, such as panic attacks, sweating, nausea, fatigue, and depression.

> If your loved one has PDD or has had any predementia symptoms such as active dreams or hallucinations, talk to the physician about changing to a drug that is safer to use with LBD, such as Sinemet.

Sinemet and other PD drugs can allow persons with Parkinson's disease to have many years of functional movement they might not otherwise have, but they can only slow the progression of PD. They cannot stop it.

Balancing the Drugs

Dopamine, the chemical that acts to control movement, has anticholinergic properties, meaning it can cause or increase dementia symptoms. Thus, when the PD drugs like Sinemet increase dopamine in the brain they also increase the chance of symptoms such as confusion and hallucinations.

> After Bill retired he began having spells when he just wasn't thinking clearly. As a nurse, I'd studied PD, and I knew that dementia was a possibility. Of course, we'd hoped he'd be one of the 50% or so who won the "PD lottery" and didn't develop dementia. No such luck. First it was just really poor decisions, but when he started having hallucinations, I made a doctor's appointment for him. His doctor decreased his PD meds and that seemed to work. The bad part was that he had to start using a walker because his mobility was so much poorer, but we could accept that better than dementia. Maybe it had been the PD meds causing Bill's dementia symptoms, we thought. Maybe we still had a chance to win the "PD lottery."
>
> —*Barbara*

One possible reason for Bill's beginning dementia symptoms was his PD medication. Sometimes lowering the dose or stopping the medication altogether will stop the dementia symptoms.

> The respite only lasted a few months before Bill started having hallucinations again. He was also having such active dreams that I moved out of our bed to protect myself from his flailing limbs. We went back to the doctor, who added Exelon, the dementia drug recommended for people with PDD. His hallucinations and his active dreams stopped, and he started thinking more clearly. I had my Bill back again—but at a cost; his mobility was much worse. I was still working, so we had to have someone come and stay with Bill. He just wasn't safe alone anymore.
>
> —*Barbara*

When decreasing the PD medications did not work, Barbara knew they had not won the "PD lottery." The Lewy bodies had traveled from Bill's motor control center to his cognition center and they, not the PD medicine, were causing the dementia. Bill's Parkinson's disease had become PDD—one of the two types of Lewy body dementia.

With the onset of PDD, Bill now had two opposing sets of symptoms to fight: his old familiar movement dysfunctions and these new dementia symptoms. These groups of symptoms are at opposite poles when it comes to treatment. Think of them as being situated with one at each end of a treatment balance board, like a teeter-totter. Drugs that improve one group of symptoms are likely to make the other group of symptoms worse: the drugs used to treat the motor symptoms will cause dementia symptoms to appear or increase, and those that treat dementia will cause adverse motor symptoms to appear or increase. This important aspect of PDD will be discussed further in Chapter 8.

With PD, one's role as caregiver is mostly physical. My experience with my sister Lucille, who had PD, is a good example. I helped her in and out of bed and wrote checks for her when the characteristic small writing made it too difficult for her. In addition, her balance was so poor that she used a walker. However, her mental abilities were still good, and I did not have to make decisions for her.

When PDD sets in the relationship between caregiver and loved one must change. This period of transition is a good time to make some decisions together, such as what to do now and in the future.

> When we found out that Bill had PDD, we sat down and discussed how we wanted to deal with it. We knew we'd have choices to make about medications and agreed that we'd choose cognition over mobility whenever we could. We also discussed other issues, such as physical care options. Later, I was so glad we'd done that because when I had to make these decisions myself, I knew they were in line with what Bill would have wanted.
>
> *— Barbara*

Caregivers repeatedly voice agreement with Barbara and Bill's decision to choose cognition over mobility. Most say they are willing to do extra work to have their loved one present in mind as well as body, or at least as present as possible.

Decisions such as the one Barbara and Bill made are not one-time decisions. They must be made repeatedly throughout a family's journey with this disease. Because Barbara knew Bill's feelings about this matter, her decisions later on, when he was increasingly less able to participate, were easier for her to make and easier for Bill to accept.

As the dementia increases, your job as decision maker will also increase, just as Barbara's job did. Although the doctors will always be a part of the decision-making process, in the end, it is up to the family to make choices—not just the choice between cognition and mobility, but many others as well, such as when it is time to give up trying to keep your loved one at home. Look for sources of support from family members, group members, or friends. Otherwise, this can be a lonely, sometimes scary job.

A person with Parkinson's disease with dementia:

- First has the motor symptoms of PD and then develops cognitive symptoms, and
- Will usually experience early warning signs, such as active dreams or hallucinations, before there are any cognitive dysfunctions.

Motor Symptoms That Start After Dementia

If the motor dysfunctions occur after the dementia, as in someone with dementia with Lewy bodies, we call these symptoms *parkinsonism*. A common theory is that Lewy bodies migrate outward from the motor center to the cerebral cortex. If this is so, Lewy bodies that start in the cerebral cortex (as with DLB) would be less likely to migrate inward and cause movement dysfunctions. We do know that when motor dysfunctions first appear after the advent of dementia they are more likely to be caused by cognition medication than by Lewy bodies.

After David had been on Aricept for a while, he started having periods when he couldn't keep his hands from shaking. His neurologist tried giving him a small dose of Sinemet. That stopped the shaking, but David went back to having hallucinations. Of course we stopped the Sinemet. Now, his doctor is still trying to find the right combination of dementia meds for him.

—*Marie*

David, who has early-onset DLB, had developed a tremor, a motor symptom often seen with Parkinson's disease. Because the tremor showed up after David started taking donepezil (Aricept), it was likely that the cognition drug caused the tremors. However, rather than return to the trial and error needed to find a different mixture of cognition drugs, his doctor tried for an "easier" answer first. He added the PD drug Sinemet. When that did not work, his doctor went back to trying out different dementia drug combinations. David and his doctor may have to try several times before they find the best solution.

Balancing the Drugs

The balance issue is not quite so difficult for the person with DLB. Without the need for drugs to control motor functions as well as cognition, there are not as many choices to make. It is mostly a matter of trying out different cognition medications and dose levels to see which one causes the least motor dysfunction while still treating the dementia.

> *Parkinsonism:* Motor symptoms that occur after a person has been diagnosed with DLB and that are usually brought on by dementia medications.

Even though David has DLB, he must deal with some movement issues. A side effect of all dementia drugs is that they can also cause motor dysfunctions. David and Marie may have to make the same choice between mobility and cognition that Barbara and Bill had to make. For now, David may have to settle for a certain amount of tremor to get the cognitive improvement he wants. However, motor symptoms caused by cognition medications tend to be less severe than those caused by Lewy bodies, and they are also temporary—once the drug is out of the system, the motor dysfunctions go away.

6

Sleep Disorders and Lewy Body Dementia

Almost all people with Lewy body dementia (LBD) will have had some kind of sleep disorder before they develop dementia symptoms. And, of course, the sleep issues continue after dementia shows up.

The two most prominent sleep-related problems appear to be at odds with each other: rapid eye movement (REM) sleep behavior disorder (RBD) disturbs sleep and excessive daytime sleeping (EDS) causes too much sleep. However, both are easily within the realm of elements common to LBD: vivid-but-not-real experiences and a general slowing down of all body functions. The literature occasionally mentions insomnia as a symptom, but caregivers seldom do. Usually, interrupted nighttime sleep is caused by the active dreams of RBD or the irritations of restless leg syndrome (RLS), another sleep disorder common with Lewy body dementia.

General Treatment

Maintaining good sleeping habits promotes better sleep for people in general and serves to decrease LBD-related sleep disturbances.

- Try a fixed routine that includes:
  - A comfortable bedroom and bed;
  - A regular bedtime with a comforting bedtime routine;
  - Regular exercise, but not right before bedtime; and
  - Little food and no coffee several hours before bedtime.
- Limit alcohol and especially do not give any at bedtime.
- Arrange with the physician to give your loved one the largest doses of drugs that may cause drowsiness, such as

medications against acting out, just before bedtime and drugs for alertness, such as modafinil (Provigil), in the morning.

- Review the list of possible stressors in Chapter 9, and eliminate as many as possible from your loved one's routine.

- Most sleep aids are contraindicated, meaning it is inadvisable to use them because of an underlying condition, in this case, LBD (see Chapter 8 for a discussion of sleep aids, their dangers, and some possible alternatives).

REM Sleep Behavior Disorder

What Is RBD?

During normal dreams, or rapid eye movement (REM) sleep, the eyes move so much that they make the eyelids flutter. However, the rest of a normally functioning body is temporarily paralyzed, which allows the body to remain at rest during even the most active dream sequences. REM sleep behavior disorder is a brain dysfunction that removes this restriction and allows movement. When people with RBD dream, they act out their dreams, talking and moving their limbs and sometimes becoming quite violent. RBD is also called "active dreaming." These dreams, like hallucinations and delusions, are behavioral symptoms of LBD.

> Anique would wave her arms and thrash her legs about and hold long conversations. I remember wondering what the other person was saying. Of course, she was fluent in three languages, and so sometimes I couldn't understand her.
>
> —Jim

RBD is so common with Lewy body dementia that it is a defining symptom. It can start years before any sign of cognitive dysfunction. At least 50% of people who have active dreams will go on to develop LBD. If an active dreamer also has Parkinson's disease (PD), the percentage is even greater.

> Anique's active dreams began years before she had any signs of dementia, and we never connected the two. Why would we? She was still thinking clearly and wasn't even forgetting anything when they started.
>
> —Jim

A person may have RBD and not know it. Because dreamers seldom remember anything about their behavior upon awakening, identifying when their active dreams began requires a witness. I often wondered if my sister Lucille, who had PD, had active dreams. However, my sister never married and with only her cat as a sleeping companion, there was no one to say.

Not all people who talk or walk in their sleep have RBD. Sleep-talking and sleepwalking can also occur during non-REM sleep, when the person is asleep but not dreaming. These behaviors are especially common with children and are not predictive of Lewy body dementia.

> If the active dreams become more frequent and intense, look for increased stress as a cause.

Active Dreams as a Warning Sign

Because RBD often starts years before any other LBD symptoms, it is considered a predictor of the disease. A person who has active dreams but no signs of dementia should consider the dreams a warning. Remember that a "defining event" of extreme stress, such as surgery, illness, or a severe reaction to certain medications may increase already-present dementia symptoms. It can also initiate dementia symptoms in someone who, up to that point, has apparently been dementia free. Therefore, anyone with active dreams should avoid optional surgeries and drugs that are considered dangerous for someone with LBD every bit as carefully as someone who already has dementia.

> We never connected Peter's active dreams with his dementia or reported them to his doctor. And until this last surgery after Peter fell and broke his hip, no doctors ever asked me if Peter had active dreams.
>
> —*Jenny*

People with RBD who are contemplating surgery should tell their doctor about the dreams. An LBD-savvy physician will ask, but you do not have to wait for the question before sharing this information, and if the doctor is not concerned, consider a different doctor. Share this information with your friends and relatives and to everyone you know. Many people, like Jim and Anique, did not know the dreams were important until it was too late.

Today, you can find information about LBD and the importance of knowing its predictors in magazines and other places besides your doctor's office. A list of resources can also be found in the back of this book.

> My mom's dentist told her that if she had some major dental surgery, her teeth would look straighter and be easier to clean. She was about to do it when I read an article about LBD in a magazine. It mentioned that RBD was a very common precursor of LBD. My dad has been complaining about Mom's thrashing about in bed for a couple of years. I told Mom, and she decided not to have the surgery. "I sure do hope I'm one of the 50% that isn't going to have dementia, but I'm not going to push my luck," is what she said.
>
> —*Allison*

Allison's mom may have avoided an early onset of dementia. This is one of those times when a surgery is optional and the choice between prettier teeth and possible dementia was a comparatively easy one to make.

Treatment

- Follow the general treatment suggestions at the start of this chapter.
- Specific treatment for RBD is the same as it is for other behavioral symptoms (see Chapter 9).

Safety

Safety can be an issue with RBD. The active dreamer sometimes moves around so much that he falls out of bed, or he can get up and wander around in his dreams, bumping into furniture or falling. When limbs thrash about, a bed partner can easily be hit.

> Once I woke up because Anique was trying to hit me. I grabbed her wrists and held them for a few moments, and then she relaxed. When I let go she rolled over and went into a peaceful sleep.
>
> —*Jim*

Jim was much bigger than Anique, so it was easy for him to stop her. Other caregivers report instances where they have not been as fortunate. Black eyes and other bruises are not uncommon.

In the morning, I teased Anique about "beating me up," but she didn't remember the incident at all. Not long after that, we exchanged our queen-sized bed for twin beds.

—Jim

Active dreamers seldom remember their attacks, or what they were dreaming at the time. Jim's solution of moving into separate beds is one many caregivers resort to. This allows them to get much-needed sleep without being continually on guard against sudden "attacks."

Other safeguards might include:

- Moving any objects that could cause injury away from the bedside and padding those that are too heavy or impractical to move;
- Padding the headboard;
- Moving the bed away from windows, and/or blocking them with an immovable object, such as a heavy dresser; and
- Having well-carpeted floors or placing padding next to the bed.

- REM sleep behavior disorder, or active dreams, can begin years before any sign of cognitive dysfunction.
- Treat active dreams the same as any other acting-out behavior, and keep the dreamer's sleeping environment safe to prevent injury.

Restless Leg Syndrome

Although sometimes confused with RBD, restless leg syndrome[1] is not the same thing. Although it does often occur at night, it has nothing to do with dreams. In fact, RLS is not even an LBD-related dysfunction. Dementia drugs have no effect on it, and a person with RLS has the same chance as anyone in the general public of eventually developing LBD. However, this annoying syndrome is common with many neurological disorders, including Lewy body dementia.

Symptoms of RLS (a) include strong urges to move in order to stop painful or odd sensations, (b) can occur while the patient is asleep or awake, and (c) may begin years before any symptoms connected with dementia occur.

Treatment

There is no cure for restless leg syndrome, and many of the drugs normally used to relieve it are not recommended for use with LBD.

- Drugs sometimes used for RLS but not recommended for anyone with Lewy body dementia include the following:
  - *Benzodiazepines:* Because these drugs are addictive, they should not be used for ongoing problems.
  - *Opiates:* These drugs are well-known for being addictive, and the small doses tolerated by a person with Lewy body dementia may not be effective against RLS.
  - *Anticonvulsants:* These drugs, including gabapentin (Neurontin), have side effects that include excessive sleepiness and gait problems.
  - *Quinine:* Although recommended for leg cramps by some LBD caregivers, research has not shown this drug to be of great help for restless leg syndrome. In addition, it can have serious adverse reactions, including death.[2]
- Drugs that may be useful and safe when monitored carefully include the following:
  - *Ropinirole (Requip) and pramipexole (Mirapex):* Approved by the Federal Drug Administration for moderate to severe RLS, both drugs are in the same drug family as those used to treat Parkinson's disease. Although they may decrease cognition and increase behavioral symptoms, the effect is temporary. Therefore, they are likely safe to try with careful monitoring.
  - *Iron supplements:* RLS may occur because of a lack of iron, but because too much iron can cause damage, you should get a doctor's approval before using it.
  - *Over-the-counter (OTC) pain relievers:* These may be safe but are effective only for mild RLS. Always check with the physician before giving your loved one OTC drugs.

○ *Nonbenzodiazepine sedatives:* Among others, trazodone (Desyrel) or divalproex (Depakote) may be prescribed for RLS that occurs most frequently at bedtime. Of all the drug choices, these may be the best selection for someone with Lewy body dementia, but they are not useful for daytime RLS.

Dementia drugs do not have any effect on RLS.

The best all-around interventions to restless leg syndrome are generally caregiver driven. The following may limit or prevent RLS:

- *Ensuring regular exercise:* The more movement, the less RLS. The exercise should not be extreme and should be done well before bedtime.
- *Applying pressure:* During the day, use pantyhose or wrap the legs in Ace bandages.
- *Reducing caffeine, alcohol, and tobacco use:* This is particularly important in the evening.

To stop an RLS episode, try:

- *Moving:* Move the affected limb(s) for a few minutes. Restless leg syndrome is usually relieved by movement.
- *Applying heat or cold:* A bath or foot soak may help.
- *Using a pillow:* Place your loved one on his side with a pillow between his knees. Make him as comfortable as possible.

Mom sometimes complains about RLS. Usually she's in bed and we don't want to get her up unless we have to so I've found the best thing to do for her is to massage her legs. If that doesn't work, then we go ahead and get her up and let her move around—a walk to the bathroom and back usually does the job. When I put her back to bed, I make sure she is really comfortable, with as little pressure as possible on her legs.

—*Marion, daughter of Clara*

Marion recognizes that hands-on remedies are safer than the medications, and often they are just as successful. She could also take some preventative steps if the RLS occurs very often, like having her mother wear support hose and do more exercise during the day.

Restless leg syndrome is:

- Not an LBD-related symptom like RBD,
- Not affected by dementia drugs, and
- Not a predictor of Lewy body dementia.

The drugs that treat RLS either are not recommended or have some serious drawbacks, making caregiver-driven interventions such as exercise and massage the most effective remedies.

Excessive Daytime Sleeping

Excessive daytime sleeping is a symptom of the slowing down of the brain. Although it is also associated with other neurological diseases, including Alzheimer's and Parkinson's, it is usually present with LBD, especially in advanced stages.

Jerome used to get up at about nine AM, have breakfast with me, and then be awake until after lunch. He'd nap for a couple of hours in the afternoon, and then he was in bed for the night—I hoped—by eight PM. If he had a bad night, with active dreams, he might wake up several times, but that didn't seem to make much difference in his daytime schedule. Over the last few months, I've noticed that he's gradually sleeping more and more during the day. This last week, he napped in the morning as well as the afternoon, and I can't keep him up much later than seven.

—*Cathy*

Jerome's increased sleeping is par for the course. As the LBD progresses, a person just seems to need more sleep. He may appear compelled to nap repeatedly during the day, even falling asleep at inappropriate times, such as during meals. Sleeping well at night does not keep a person with EDS from feeling exhausted or drowsy during the day.

Dad sleeps a lot, but Mom says that when I come to visit he sleeps much less. He loves going over his old photos with me, and I know he's often missed his afternoon nap so he could keep on telling me about the people in those photos. Maybe he doesn't need as much sleep as Mom thinks he does. Maybe he's just bored.

—*Kyla, daughter of Ed*

Although excessive daytime sleeping is an involuntary behavior, it may appear that Ed can make himself stay awake when he wants to. He may occasionally stay awake when something grabs his interest or while doing something especially enjoyable. However, he cannot control this anymore than he can control the *showtime* aspect of fluctuating cognition. (See Chapter 4)

Not all physicians, even those who specialize in the elderly, appear to be aware of how common EDS is with LBD.

When I told my mother's geriatric neuropsychiatrist about Mom's fifteen hours of sleep every night, he suspected overmedication and reduced her drugs. That caused Mom to start sleeping poorly at night. I did an informal survey of my online support group and found that, with daytime naps included, 15 hours of sleep per day was not abnormal for our loved ones. I've long thought that illness in and of itself requires extra sleep, and certainly the efforts our loved ones put out to walk without falling, eat without choking, and try their darndest to be normal must demand extra rest too.

—Marion, daughter of Clara

Marion has a point. Add to this the general slowing-down effect of LBD and it is no surprise that LBD patients spend much of their time sleeping.

Peter seems so tired lately—more so than usual. He's sleeping almost 20 hours a day now. We had a busy schedule with our sons both coming to visit last week, so maybe he is just catching up. Should I be worried?

—Jenny

Being fatigued is part of LBD, and sleeping will gradually take up more and more of a person's day. After a period of *showtime* alertness for his visiting family, it is reasonable to expect Peter to sleep more than usual for a day or so. However, it has been a week now, and he is still sleeping most of the day. Caregivers warn that sleeping for more than 20 hours is often a sign that the end may be near.

As a general rule, daytime sleeping will occur whether your loved one has a good night's sleep or not. However, caregivers report that controlling RBD activity will reduce daytime sleeping, especially if the active dreaming was traumatic.

Jake was in a lot of battles during his time in service. His dreams are usually very scary, and I can tell from his shouting that he is back there again.

—Norma

Jake was refighting his war experiences and, although he was asleep, he was not getting much rest. If the dreams take up a large part of the night, they are probably spilling over into normal deep sleep time, robbing him not only of restful dreamtime but also of the time when his brain should be transferring information from short to long-term memory. Thus, he may be "catching up" during daytime sleeping.[3]

Treatment

- *Dementia drugs:* As with all LBD-related dysfunctions these may help maintain daytime alertness, but eventually they become less effective.
- *Modafinil (Provigil):* This drug is approved for sleep disturbances and has worked well to limit sleep for some people with LBD. Even though it is a stimulant, it does not have the anxiety-producing side effects that other stimulants have. Provigil may also improve cognition.

When Jake's doctor prescribed Provigil for his excessive sleeping, he said it might improve his cognition and even make him have fewer active dreams. Wow! A wonder drug! Well, it did make a difference with his sleeping and I think his dreams have been less violent. The doctor said we could use Seroquel for the dreams if we needed to, but so far the dementia meds and the Provigil have been enough.

—Norma

Provigil and the dementia drugs are both considered safer drugs than the atypical antipsychotics, such as quetiapine (Seroquel), used to decrease acting-out behavior. As long as they work to decrease the EDS, there is no need to add another drug. However, as the dementia progresses, Seroquel or some similar additional drug may be useful.

As with other LBD-related symptoms, caregiver-based intervention is the best deterrent of excessive daytime sleeping.

- In addition to the general treatment suggestions at the start of this chapter, lowering stress can often help.

- If your loved one has PDD, his Parkinson's medications may cause excessive sleeping.

- Caregiving can be a very demanding job. Take the time while your loved one is sleeping to do something for yourself. Go play a game, read, do your fingernails, or even take a nap. Keeping yourself balanced will make you a better caregiver.

Although a person with excessive daytime sleeping can sometimes manage to stay awake and alert during periods of special interest, EDS is involuntary and will increase with the progress of LBD.

Insomnia

The literature occasionally mentions insomnia as a symptom of LBD, but caregivers seldom do. Because LBD is mostly a slowing of all one's facilities, it is understandable that insomnia is not common. In fact, too much sleep, as with excessive daytime sleep, is more likely. However, people with LBD may be unable to sleep for various reasons resulting from LBD-related issues:

- Circadian rhythms may be disrupted by problems such as EDS or active dreams.

- Sleep may be interrupted by bad dreams or urinary problems.

- Once awake, the individual may not realize that it is night and wander instead of going back to sleep.

- Some medications given in the evening can cause wakefulness.

Most sleep aid drugs are contraindicated for anyone with LBD (see Chapter 9 for a discussion of sleep aids, their dangers, and some safer alternatives). All of the suggestions under "General Treatment" section at the beginning of this chapter may help your loved one's insomnia.

Primary caregivers are very susceptible to insomnia. Although their charges may manage to fall asleep after an interruption, the caregivers may not because they had to be more alert to provide help and maintain safety. Once their loved one is resettled, caregivers often find sleep elusive. This leads to fatigue-related irritability that is likely to increase their loved one's acting out, which in turn increases the caregiver's frustration, causing a vicious cycle unless the sleep problems of both individuals are addressed.

> Jake's dreams wake me up more than they do him. And then I have an awful time getting back to sleep. When Jake's dreams were getting worse and worse, I talked to our health aide and she suggested that when I've had a bad night, I take a nap while she is here. I complain about Jake and she wants to fix me! But it worked. With me happier and easier to live with, Jake is having fewer active dreams.
>
> —*Norma*

Most caregivers hesitate to take sleeping pills because they want to be able to wake up easily if their loved one needs them. Consider these drug-free interventions to get a good night's sleep.

- Presleep rituals can help you too. Give yourself some special alone time once you have your loved one tucked in for the night. An hour of reading a favorite book followed by a nice cup of chamomile tea may help you sleep.
- Take "power naps" during the day. You will be surprised at how a few minutes here, a half hour there, will help you feel more rested. If you can take advantage of the presence of a home care worker or a family member's visit to take a nap, do it.
- If you sleep separately from your loved one and cannot sleep soundly for fear he will need you, use an electronic baby monitor to warn you if he wakes up.

Finally, do not hesitate to ask for help. Perhaps you can ask a relative or friend come and sit with your loved one for an hour while you escape to the bedroom for a nap. You will work better with your loved one if you are rested.

7

What Are Perceptual Dysfunctions?

The symptoms in this chapter are called *psychological, psychiatric,* or even *psychotic.* Many of these symptoms do lead to disruptive behavior, similar to that of someone with the kind of problems usually treated by a psychiatrist. However, most psychiatric drugs can cause dangerous side effects when used to treat Lewy body dementia (LBD) symptoms. Therefore, Jim and I prefer to avoid psychiatric terms and call these symptoms *"perceptual dysfunctions."* This term is accurate; people with these dysfunctions view their world differently than other people do.

Perception is the interpretation of what we:

- See with our eyes. I might see a wavy line and interpret it as writing or an outline of a face.
- Hear with our ears. I might hear a boom and interpret it as a drumbeat or an explosion.
- Feel with our skin. I might touch a surface and interpret it as hot or cold.
- Taste with our tongue. I might take a bite of food and interpret it as salty or sweet.
- Smell with our nose. I might sniff the air and interpret the odor I smell as perfume or garlic.

Delusions come about when we believe something that is false to be true. This is a *mental* misperception, an error of thinking. However, all perceptions depend on our thinking skills and our recall of past experiences to make judgments about what our sensory organs tell us.

LBD damages the interpretation process so that a person will:

- Perceive objects that are not there (hallucinations),
- Interpret objects that are there as something they are not (illusions),
- Perceive objects not to be where they are (poor depth perception), or
- Believe false information to be true (delusions or mental misperceptions).

As with all LBD symptoms, those involving perceptions may come and go. Sometimes your loved ones will perceive things quite clearly. At other times, they may not. This is simply a part of the fluctuating cognition discussed in Chapter 4.

Stress is a major factor in perceptual dysfunction. It increases the likelihood of these symptoms and decreases your loved one's ability to deal with them when they do occur. This is examined further in Chapter 9 when I discuss behavior management.

General Treatment

Medical treatment for all perceptual dysfunctions is the same: none, unless the perceptions are disruptive, in which case as little intervention as possible should be used. I have mentioned drug sensitivities as a major issue for a person with LBD. The drugs most commonly used to treat acting out in the general population are, sadly, also the drugs most likely to cause problems for someone with LBD. We discuss these drugs, along with safer alternatives, in Chapter 8. Because of the many issues surrounding the proper use of medications for people with LBD, behavior management, discussed in Chapter 9, should be the treatment of choice whenever possible. Even if medication is required, behavior management will usually decrease the amount needed.

Perceptual dysfunctions:

- Can come and go with the fluctuating cognition of LBD;
- Are often made worse by stress; and
- Seldom need treatment unless they are disruptive, and even then, behavior management techniques should be tried prior to medication.

Hallucinations

Vivid, well-formed visual *hallucinations*, or seeing something that is not there, are a defining symptom of Lewy body dementia. LBD hallucinations tend to be more realistic than those experienced by people with Alzheimer's disease (AD), and those in early and mid-stage dementia are usually benign. Many of these hallucinations are about children.

> We'd be sitting in the living room and Anique would whisper to me, "There are children coming out from behind the TV set." I'd get up and go look behind the set and tell her, "Well, I don't see any door here, but I'll send the kids home." And then I'd make shooing motions and say, "Come on kids, time to go home," and usher them out the front door. That always satisfied her.
>
> —*Jim*

LBD hallucinations often reoccur, another dissimilarity with AD-related hallucinations. Anique saw the kids about once a week and had other less frequent recurring hallucinations. Jim says they never bothered her; she just wanted him to know she saw them. Hallucinations related to LBD may show up early in the progression of the disease, whereas those related to AD seldom appear until the end stages. The two dementias do tend to overlap, so the appearance of hallucinations, even late in the disease, may actually be caused by some Lewy bodies in the brain.

Sometimes hallucinations are the earliest noticeable symptom of LBD.

> Hallucinations are what triggered us into taking Hilda to a doctor to see what was wrong. She kept seeing things I couldn't see. She wasn't scared, but she sure was upset that I couldn't see them. They were so clear to her!
>
> —*Barney*

The doctor found that Hilda, age 62, also had some other mild dementia symptoms, including the organizational problems she had been having at work. He diagnosed her with probable LBD and offered to put her on dementia medications. Although the hallucinations were not scary, the couple chose to wait until she had some other, more distressing problems. This is a personal choice. Others may want to start medications immediately in hopes of slowing down the dementia.

People with Parkinson's disease (PD) may also develop hallucinations. My sister Lucille, who had PD, had a dearly beloved cat named Pansy. When she developed terminal cancer and became too ill to take care of Pansy, Lucille gave the cat away. She occasionally talked about how Pansy was visiting. She knew the cat was not real, but the hallucination did not distress her; in fact, she seemed to enjoy the visits.

Dogs and other small animals, along with children, such as those that Anique saw, are among the most common kinds of hallucinations. Lucille's visiting cat was likely an early sign that, if she had lived long enough, her PD would have eventually turned into Parkinson's disease dementia (PDD).

Long-gone relatives and once-known friends are also common candidates for visits via hallucinations.

> Mom has hallucinations now and then. Yesterday, she "saw" Aunt Mabel in the living room. Aunt Mabel passed on 10 years ago. I asked her if Aunt Mabel was disturbing her, and Mom said no, she's just sitting there.
>
> —*Marion, daughter of Clara*

Notice that in Clara's hallucination Aunt Mabel just sat there. She did not talk. Caregivers of people with LBD tell us that the people in their hallucinations seldom, if ever, talk. They are just there. This is one difference between the LBD hallucinations and those experienced by people with psychiatric diseases, whose hallucinations often involve voices.

Although most LBD hallucinations are not frightening, that can change when they are combined with some sort of stress, such as a violent TV program, memories of distressful past experiences, or even an infection.

> Before his hip surgery, Peter had mild hallucinations, but afterwards he started dreaming about his war years. Those horrid experiences along with the delusions he started having and, well, just his general confusion, made his hallucinations pretty scary for him.
>
> —*Jenny*

The hallucinations also can become much more plentiful as the disease progresses.

We live in a continual circus of small animals, people Emma used to know, and who knows what else. She's always "seeing" something. Most of the time it's harmless, and I just go with the flow. At other times, she gets frightened or angry, and then I try to distract her.

—Howard

Emma's dementia is advanced, and she is usually confused and accompanied by the creatures and people of her many hallucinations. Often, the hallucinations cross over into her delusions, which can then become scary or make her upset.

Nonvisual Hallucinations

There are several types of nonvisual hallucinations.[1] Auditory hallucinations are the most common, occurring for about one third of people with LBD.

Anique would hear a phone ring. I'd answer and no one was there. She'd hear someone knocking on the door. I'd answer that and, again, no one was there. She'd want me to go back and check, she was so sure she'd heard someone.

—Jim

Others may have "presence" hallucinations, in which they have a sense that someone or something is near, but just out of sight, maybe right behind them. Taste and touch hallucinations are comparatively rare. Olfactory (smell-related) hallucinations also are uncommon. However, they can be informally predictive of PDD.

Ten years ago, not long after Mom was diagnosed with PD, she lost her sense of smell. And then about 3 years ago, she began complaining of a "stinky aroma" in the house and kept bugging me to find what was causing it. I couldn't smell anything, but I checked all the usual places—garbage cans and so on. I never did find anything. A couple of months later, Mom was diagnosed with PDD.

—Marion, daughter of Clara

An impaired sense of smell is an early indicator of PD, and Clara's unwelcome "aroma" was a hallucination—and an early indicator of eventual dementia. Caregivers of people with PDD occasionally report that when they think back, their loved one's first sign of dementia was smell hallucinations like Clara's.

Coping with hallucinations is usually a matter of ignoring them— or, if they become scary, a matter of providing a distraction. If the hallucination is not scary or harmful, you can usually let it run its course.

Hallucinations: The perception of something that is not real. They seldom need treatment.

Illusions

Unlike hallucinations, in which the person sees something that is not there, an *illusion* is a real object that the person sees incorrectly. Illusions can be general, or they can be expressed as poor depth perception or poor hand–eye coordination.

An example of a general illusion is when a person "sees" a small animal instead of the shoebox that is really there.

> I have this black fluffy blob that shows up pretty often. I call it my pet dog. He's off over there right now. I know he isn't real, but he keeps me company.
> —*Terry, who has PD*

When Terry sees something peripherally, such as a small box or a ball, his damaged perceptions turn it into a "black fluffy blob." Terry, who still has very good cognitive function, deals with this reoccurring illusion by making it his pet—and therefore a comforting presence instead of an annoying one. Terry's "pet" is a predictor that he is likely to develop PDD. However, illusions can also be scary. Anique was frightened when she saw the TV on the airplane and interpreted it as fire. Jim was able to calm her down by explaining what it really was. At other times, he had less success.

> One evening, Anique and I were standing on a hotel balcony in Europe. She pointed toward a brightly lit entertainment park just down the street and cried, "Fire!" That time, I don't think I really convinced her it wasn't a fire. She wouldn't go out on the balcony the rest of the time we were there.
> —*Jim*

Anique's dementia was still mild enough that she could usually accept Jim's explanation. However, the lights at night were scary enough that she did not want to see them anymore, even if she knew Jim was right about there being no fire. Illusions can be triggered by the same stimuli repeatedly. For instance, whenever Anique saw a flashing light she could not identify, she saw "fire."

> Objects your loved one cannot easily identify, such as something seen peripherally, may trigger a general illusion.

Poor Depth Perception

Poor depth perception is a type of illusion in which people misjudge distances between themselves and objects or other people. People with this dysfunction often perceive a change in floor texture as a change in height.

I notice that David is beginning to lift his feet as though he's climbing stairs when he goes from our vinyl kitchen floor to our carpeted living room.

—Marie

David is starting to have problems with depth perception. He perceives the carpet to be higher than the vinyl floor and automatically lifts his feet when he goes from one to the other. Caregivers say that they seldom see their loved ones step down—they usually step up.

Hilda was always so light on her feet, but now she's gotten clumsy. She stumbles, and once she even fell. The doctor is suggesting a cane, but she's not willing yet.

—Barney

In Hilda's case, "clumsy" means that she is misjudging distances and stumbling over obstacles when she perceives the way is clear. Hilda has early dementia with Lewy bodies (DLB), the kind of Lewy body dementia that involves fewer motor problems, and she has no trouble walking. That makes it even harder for her to change her perception of herself from someone who is "light on my feet" to someone who needs a cane to keep from falling. Ideally, Hilda will make the transition to using a cane before she falls again and seriously injures herself.

Poor Hand–Eye Coordination

Hand–eye coordination is a special type of depth perception: the ability to connect one's hand with a seen goal, for example, reaching out and grasping a cup or copying a simple drawing. People with LBD tend to have more difficulty with this than do people with other dementias. Because of this, many neurologists use a clock drawing test to help with diagnosis. Points are given for correctness, and the lower the score, the higher the probability of LBD.

When Jake's neurologist had him draw a clock (see Figure 7.1), he lost points for the irregular circle, having the numbers bunched in the middle, the thirteenth number, and the placement of the hands. Jake's score indicated an increased probability of LBD.

Poor hand–eye coordination shows up in everyday living tasks.

Mom sometimes has trouble feeding herself. When she reaches for the food on her plate, it isn't where her eyes tell her it is. She stabs her fork into the table beside her plate, or on the other side of the plate, and once she even knocked over her water glass.

—Marion, daughter of Clara

Notice that Marion says her mom has problems only sometimes. LBD's fluctuating cognition means Marion never knows if her mom will need help with her eating or not.

I've started filling Jake's coffee cup only about half full. He doesn't shake; it's just that he misjudges where the cup is and tips it over when he reaches for it. And once when I gave him an ice cream cone he smashed the ice cream onto his glasses instead of getting it to his mouth.

—Norma

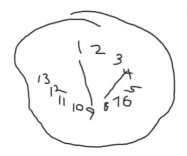

Figure 7.1　Simulated results of Jake's clock test.

Like Clara, Jake is displaying failing hand–eye coordination. He might also have trouble connecting if someone offered to shake his hand, and doing jigsaw puzzles would be practically impossible unless he used huge pieces.

Systemized Delusions

A *delusion* is a false, often-paranoid belief that is a mental rather than sensory misperception. These false beliefs can appear alone, but most often they can accompany dreams, hallucinations, media stories, or actual events. Unlike the fairly simple delusions of AD, LBD delusions tend to be persistent and systemized; that is, the person builds them over time into a complicated story or drama.

> Every morning for about a week, my wife, Janet, would see nonexistent workers come into our apartment and go down into our nonexistent basement by way of a nonexistent door under our living room sofa. In the evening, her workers returned the same way they went in. Once, she offered them drinks before they left to go home. That same evening, we went for a drive and got stuck in a traffic jam caused by a bad accident. As we drove by the wrecked car, Janet became hysterical. She was sure that the car belonged to a worker from under our sofa. Therefore, in her mind, she had caused the accident by giving the guy a drink.
>
> —*John*

Janet's delusion included hallucinations and real life events. She had developed it into an involved story, in which she was a player. Likewise, people can incorporate violent scenes from TV programs into their delusions.

> I've learned to monitor what Mom watches on TV. When I can get her to watch something besides her favorite crime shows, her delusions and hallucinations aren't nearly as disturbing.
>
> —*Marion, daughter of Clara*

An LBD-fogged brain has difficulty telling reality from fiction. Any highly active, violent, or emotional show can become fodder for delusions mixed with hallucinations or active dreams—not that a person needs extra fodder. Some delusions appear all by themselves.

Peter had this weird delusion for awhile where he was convinced that I wasn't his wife; I was a look-alike imposter. "You can't fool me," he'd say and turn his head away and not look at me at all. We've been married for 40 years. Even when I knew it was the disease and not him, it made me feel so sad when he rejected me.

—*Jenny*

Peter was experiencing Capgras syndrome, which causes a person to become convinced that someone close is a look-alike imposter. If, like Peter, the person is married, the imposter is usually the spouse.

The other day, my Harry got really upset and told me I was an imposter. I told my support group about it, and someone in the group suggested something that sounded kind of silly. Oh, well, I thought, anything is worth a try. And so the next time Harry told me he knew I was just someone who looked like his wife, I turned and walked out of the room. And then I came back minute later, slapping my hands together, you know, in the way that means, "I got that done!" And I said, "Well, I got rid of her. How are you, dear?" It worked! This time my Harry knew it was really me.

—*Nell*

Caregivers warn that Nell's solution does not always work, of course. You may have to just wait for time to do its work. The delusion will eventually go away, although caregivers report that it can last for several weeks.

> Capgras syndrome is named after the French psychiatrist Joseph Capgras, who first described this systemized delusion in 1923. It is most common with schizophrenia but also occurs in some forms of dementia, particularly LBD.

Delusions may cause your loved one to become angry, or frightened, which may bring on combativeness or other acting-out behavior. These can be more disruptive than sensory misperceptions alone, especially when they are combined with hallucinations or other stressors. At such times, when your loved one is out of control, medical treatment may be needed. Then, once he is calmer, you can often use behavior management techniques to maintain safety.

Systemized delusions are mental misperceptions developed into complicated dramas that can last for weeks. They are often combined with hallucinations, active dreams, media stories, or real events and may evolve and change with time and the addition of new information.

As LBD advances, your loved one will likely have increasing perceptual dysfunctions. The kind varies from person to person. No one's LBD is expressed in the same way. Although behavior management can help you to decrease these behaviors, this disease is progressive, and eventually your loved one may need medication not just as an emergency measure but on a regular basis.

8

Drug Sensitivities and Adverse Reactions

"Which drugs are safe? Which drugs aren't, and why?"

There are no definite answers to these questions because every person with Lewy body dementia (LBD) responds differently to different medications. First, consult a doctor about any drugs that you are taking or are thinking about having your loved one take. Always remember to disclose to your doctor not only the prescription drugs but also all over-the-counter (OTC) medications, vitamins, and herbal supplements your loved one is taking.

No one knows how an individual with LBD will respond to any drug until he has tried it. He may be so sensitive to the drug that a normal dose acts as an overdose, he may respond to the drug with additional unwanted symptoms, or he may be able to tolerate well a drug that many others with LBD cannot. Trial and error is normally the method a physician uses to find the most effective drugs for someone with LBD. However, there are some drugs even one dose of which can cause serious and perhaps permanent adverse side effects.

This confusing and occasionally devastating response to drugs is why Jim became so passionate about making others more aware of Lewy body dementia. In the early 2000s, when Anique was dealing with LBD, few people in the medical community had heard of the disease, let alone its sensitivity to drugs.

> Over a period of about a year, Anique went from being a functioning, active woman who "forgot a few things" as she described it, to being unable to care for herself, walk by herself, or think clearly. I lay the blame for this quick decline on

the drugs she was given, drugs that even then were known to be dangerous for someone with her symptoms.

—Jim

Although Anique had classic Lewy body dementia symptoms, she had been diagnosed with Alzheimer's disease (AD), as most people with LBD were at that time. Thus, she was prescribed certain drugs that, while generally safe for someone with Alzheimer's, can be dangerous to someone with LBD. Anique's reaction to these drugs was a textbook example of LBD drug sensitivity, but still no one in the medical community recognized this, and her special needs went unmet.

To ensure the safety of their loved ones, LBD caregivers may find it useful to become experts on the drugs their loved ones can and cannot use safely. This means learning the drugs to avoid and learning to look for the signs that something may be wrong with your loved one.

Before Anique developed LBD, I knew very little about medicine and drugs. I was a computer geek—I wasn't a doctor, and I wasn't interested in anything like that. When I had a headache, I took an aspirin. When I had a cough, I took some cough syrup. That was about the limit of my medical knowledge. But by the time Anique died, I had become knowledgeable about many drugs, especially those that were dangerous to use with LBD. The sad thing is, I learned all of this too late to help her.

—Jim

Jim learned to recognize certain dangerous drug types or categories. He learned to read drug labels and look for active ingredients that were unsafe for Anique, as well as how these unsafe drugs work so that he could avoid other drugs with similar actions. He also learned to recognize the generic drug names that the medical community uses instead of brand names, so that he could recognize these words in medical articles and on drug labels. These are all things that caregivers can do to better educate themselves about the drugs prescribed to their loved ones.

Quick Definitions

Drug properties: A drug's potential to act a certain way. Caregivers should be concerned with properties that have a potential to cause (*a*) dementia, (*b*) motor problems, or (*c*) sedation (some drugs have dementia-causing properties).

> *Drug action:* The way a drug acts on the human body. Caregivers should be concerned with actions that cause (*a*) dementia, (*b*) motor problems, and (*c*) sedation. A drug action has a similar potential and the terms are often used interchangeably.
>
> *Desired drug effects:* What the drug is prescribed to do.
>
> *Side effects:* What a drug does other than the desired effect. Side effects can be beneficial or harmful.
>
> *Adverse drug reactions:* Unwanted or harmful side effects (e.g., the drug rivastigmine [Exelon] acts to preserve acetylcholine, which has the desired effect of decreasing dementia symptoms and may have the adverse effect of increasing motor symptoms).

Like everyone else, a person with a Lewy body disease can have other health issues. For example, my sister Lucille also had cancer. Although the LBD may be unrelated to the other illness, it must always be taken into consideration. Medications normally used for a given health issue may not be safe at all for someone with LBD, or a normal dose may be far too strong.

In fact, drugs that may cause a person with LBD to have severe adverse side effects are used to treat a wide various disorders, including psychological or perceptual problems, anxiety, sleep disorders, incontinence, depression, allergies, cold symptoms, and pain. Inhaled anesthetics, used for general surgery—and some dental procedures—can cause serious side effects.[1] These potentially dangerous drugs can be divided into (*a*) those that may cause dementia (because of anticholinergic properties), (*b*) those that may cause motor dysfunctions, and (*c*) those that may cause sedation.

Dementia drugs, that is, those that decrease dementia symptoms, work by preserving the brain chemical acetylcholine, which is important for memory, concentration, and muscle movement and control.[2] Drugs with anticholinergic properties work by decreasing acetylcholine and thus cause dementia symptoms such as confusion, agitation, and hallucinations. When a drug with anticholinergic properties is given along with a dementia drug, the dementia drug is understandably less effective.

PD drugs, that is, those that decrease motor symptoms, are anticholinergics and therefore tend to increase dementia symptoms. Conversely, drugs used to treat dementia tend to increase motor symptoms.

For anyone with Lewy body dementia, no matter which kind, there is a balance that must always be considered and maintained.

Drugs with sedative properties depress the central nervous system (CNS) to cause symptoms ranging from light drowsiness to death. Many LBD caregivers have found that a normal dose of a drug with sedative properties will act as an overdose for their loved one, causing side effects such as extreme drowsiness, confusion, hallucinations, and delusions. The side effects caused by most sedatives are transitory—that is, they go away when the drug leaves the body.

The most dangerous drugs are those with combinations of the preceding properties.

- Traditional antipsychotics combine properties causing cognitive dysfunction, motor dysfunctions, and sedation.
- Benzodiazepines are considered sedatives but have often strong dementia-causing properties as well.

Other drugs that can cause adverse side effects for someone with LBD include[3]:

- Atypical antipsychotics,
- Decongestants and antihistamines used to treat colds and allergies,
- Some antidepressants,
- Antispasmodics used to relax muscles and treat incontinence,
- Strong pain medications, and
- Inhaled surgical anesthetics.

Quick Facts

- Many drugs used with comparative safety by the general public can cause dangerous side effects for someone with LBD.
- Each person with LBD responds to drugs in his own way.
- The drugs most dangerous for someone with LBD can be divided into those that can cause side effects of:
  ○ Dementia symptoms, such as confusion and hallucinations;

- Motor dysfunctions, such as tremors or muscle constriction; and

- Heavy sedation.

• Traditional antipsychotics and benzodiazepines, which can cause more than one type of the preceding symptoms, are generally the most dangerous.

Because the list of drugs that can trigger serious LBD-related side effects is so large, it is important to be aware of each drug your loved one takes and its possible side effects and then monitor its use carefully.

If you have managed to find an LBD-savvy doctor, you can trust that he or she will know the basic drugs to avoid. Even so, if your loved one is seeing the doctor for an illness unrelated to LBD, do not assume the doctor will remember to avoid prescribing LBD-dangerous drugs. Asking will remind him or her.

When only one drug is added or changed at a time you can monitor your loved one's reactions more easily.

Doctors are very busy people, and even the most dedicated can seldom find time to keep completely current on the many diseases they treat. However, remember that although you may have more time and even more interest in researching this one disease, the doctor will have a multitude of other information that may have a bearing on what your loved one is prescribed. Therefore, play it safe. Double check, but always review any new information with your doctor.

Whenever Hilda gets a new medication, I always check it out on the Internet. There are some great Web sites that tell me about drugs in words that I can actually understand. If what I read concerns me, I call her doctor's office and talk to the nurse who is, thank goodness, very knowledgeable about LBD. I'm sure they think I am a worrywart, but Hilda is more important than what they think. Usually, the nurse is aware of what I've read and is able to calm my fears. But once, what I read was new information for her. She told the doctor and he changed the medication immediately. Just that once was worth all the other times I'd called.

—*Barney*

You can also use pharmacists as a resource. When you get the prescription filled, ask about conflicts with LBD, or with another drug. Because a pharmacists' focus are on the drugs, they often know more about them than even your doctor does.

If you can use a computer, you can do as Barney did and research the drug online. MedlinePlus and WebMD have excellent drug directories. DoublecheckMD has a good drug directory as well as an easy way to search for specific side effects, such as "anticholinergic (dementia-causing) effects" and "motor effects." If you have any questions about your findings, call the doctor with your concerns. In addition, of course, always monitor any new drug carefully and report any suspicious side effects quickly so the drug can be stopped if needed.

The following are the Internet resources for checking drugs:

MedlinePlus: http://www.nlm.nih.gov/medlineplus/druginformation.html

WebMD: http://www.webmd.com/drugs/index-drugs.aspx

DoublecheckMD: http://doublecheckmd.com/

Keep a medication log. Because every person with LBD responds to medication differently, it pays to keep a daily record of your loved one's medications with:

- Date;
- Medication;
- Amount;
- Time of day the drug is taken;
- A comments section for your loved one's reactions, if any; and
- Any unusual acting out—or a decrease of acting out.

Also include any changes in routines, such as a different mealtime or bedtime than usual. These can affect medications, too.

Because problems are most likely to occur right after a new medication is started, be sure to identify the date a new drug is started and document your loved one's reactions carefully for the first few days afterward. Such a log will greatly help the physician know what to prescribe.

Drugs That Can Increase LBD Symptoms

Traditional Antipsychotics

Of all the drugs mentioned previously, those used to treat psychological problems are the ones that generate the most concern in the LBD community. For years, these drugs, called *antipsychotics*, have been used for hallucinations and other psychotic (acting-out) behaviors, even with the elderly. Of these drugs, haloperidol (Haldol) is the only one still in general use today. Although antipsychotics generally cause few side effects for someone with Alzheimer's disease, the Food and Drug Administration (FDA) recently required a *black box warning* that using antipsychotics with elderly patients with dementia increases the risk of death. This is in addition to the risk for someone with LBD, where a single dose can cause[4]:

- A decrease of cognition, which is often permanent;
- Increased and possibly irreversible motor impairment;
- Heavy sedation; and
- Symptoms resembling neuroleptic malignant syndrome (NMS): severe fever, muscle rigidity, and breakdown of the autonomic nervous system that can lead to kidney failure and death.

The preceding list of symptoms shows that traditional antipsychotics have properties that can cause dementia-related symptoms, motor dysfunctions, and sedation. It is no wonder these drugs are not considered safe for someone with LBD.

> Once, when I took Anique to the ER for dehydration, she began hallucinating and getting agitated while they were infusing her with fluids. The ER nurse gave her Haldol. I was concerned but the nurse said I shouldn't worry—they do this all the time and it would calm her right down.
>
> —*Jim*

Stress or physical illness can bring on hallucinations, delusions, or other acting-out behaviors, such as combativeness. In 2001, most emergency rooms had standing orders to calm down disruptive patients with traditional antipsychotics. Because most of the time their patients would have Alzheimer's disease, schizophrenia, or something other than LBD, antipsychotics usually worked with few if any side effects.

> Anique did calm right down. In fact, she went into a heavy sleep and wouldn't wake up. The ER doctor admitted her to the hospital overnight for observation. "Just to be safe," he told me. When she woke up hours later in the hospital, she was holding her arms tightly against her chest with her hands clenched. I tried to help her move, but even with my help, she couldn't loosen up. The hospital doctor gave her something to relax her muscles and in about an hour she could move her arms. Then she started having hallucinations. The doctor ordered regular doses of Haldol. By the next day, her muscles were constricted again. That's when doctor stopped both the Haldol and the muscle relaxants.
>
> —*Jim*

Today, many physicians would recognize Anique's overly sedated response and her contracted arm muscles as clear signs of an LBD-related sensitivity to the Haldol and immediately stop the antipsychotic. In 2001, none of the people working with Anique knew to connect these side effects with her mild dementia. Thus, she received several doses of Haldol before the doctor finally stopped it.

Hospital emergency rooms, nursing homes, and other facilities are beginning to have some knowledge about their LBD patients' sensitivities to these drugs. However, far too many doctors and other medical personnel still do not. The Lewy Body Dementia Association (LBDA) speaks to this issue by providing a free medical alert wallet card to share with medical personnel. This card contains information written by dementia specialists about drugs that should be avoided or given with extreme care to someone with LBD.

Quick Tip

Obtain the medical alert wallet card from the LBDA by going to their Web site, clicking on "Professionals" in the top menu, and then clicking on "Order Free Patient Handouts." You must order 10 at a time, so give the rest to your doctor.

When Anique came home after several days in the hospital, her muscles were almost back to normal. However, I noticed that she was knocking over her water glass more often. And it seemed to me that she wasn't quite as sharp as she'd been before. She was definitely having more hallucinations.

—*Jim*

Although Anique's dementia was still mild, the Haldol episode did have a permanent effect. Her spilled water was evidence of decreasing hand–eye coordination. In addition, her thinking skills were less acute, and her hallucinations had increased.

My Harry developed such a bad urinary [tract] infection that I took him to the emergency room. The doctor ordered some IV antibiotics, but when the nurse came to insert the IV, Harry wouldn't let her touch him. He shouted that she was trying to kill him. So another nurse came in, and they held my poor Harry down and gave him a shot of something in his arm. When I asked what they had given him, the nurse said it was Haldol. He didn't fight them anymore and by the time they had the IV in his arm, he was fast asleep. When he woke up 2 hours later, his arms were pulled close to his body, and he was really confused. Most of the confusion went away but his arms are still contracted—and that was months ago.

—*Nell*

Like Anique, Harry fell into a heavily sedated sleep and woke up with contracted muscles and confusion. However, even though Harry had only one dose of Haldol to Anique's several, his arms remained contracted and hers did not. LBD is very fickle. It does not follow rules, and affects different people differently.

Notice that both Anique's and Harry's dementia symptoms increased after they received muscle relaxants. Most muscle relaxants have anticholinergic properties and may increase dementia symptoms.

Just one dose of a traditional antipsychotic may cause possibly permanent cognitive and/or motor dysfunctions when given to someone with LBD.

The many recent caregiver reports of incidents similar to what Anique and Harry experienced show that we must be alert when we take our loved ones to emergency rooms or other places where they may be exposed to medical personnel who do not know or understand LBD.

Although the new FDA warning about antipsychotics and elderly patients with dementia may cause emergency room staff to be more careful in their use of these drugs, we caregivers cannot count on that. Moreover, if you bring your loved one in with a problem unrelated to dementia as Jim did with Anique, or if the patient is younger than 60 years of age, the staff may not perceive that they are dealing with a patient who falls into the categories of "elderly" and/or "dementia."

Because of the seriousness of this problem, family caregivers need to be proactive. You can no longer sit back and assume that the medical staff knows best. Like your doctor, medical staff in hospitals, nursing homes, and other facilities work with many conditions. They often know less about this particular disease than those of us who live and breathe it.

> I always keep my LBDA medical alert wallet card with me so if I have to take Hilda to the ER I can show it to the staff. I also wrote a note listing all the drugs I know she shouldn't be taking. I give that to the staff at the same time I give them the card. Then, I try to cover us for next time by asking the staff to copy both documents and place them in Hilda's file.
>
> —Barney

If you are like Nell, who did not know what drugs were good or bad for Harry, you can at least carry the LBDA wallet card, which does the work for you. However, the information on the card is fairly general. Barney went one step further and itemized those specific drugs he knew were unsafe for Hilda. Because Barney is Hilda's legal guardian, his signed note in her chart makes it illegal to give these drugs without consulting him first.

However, there have been caregiver reports that such written directives were still ignored. To make more impact, some caregivers have added a sentence about suing if any of the noted medications were given without their written permission.

> Besides sharing your medical alert wallet card with hospital admitting staff, plan to stay with your loved ones for most of the first day, or until they are in a hospital or care facility so that you can personally share LBD-related information with personnel on all shifts.

Atypical Antipsychotics

Some drugs, called *atypical antipsychotics*, may decrease acting-out behaviors, hallucinations, or other LBD-related behaviors with fewer side effects than those caused by the traditional antipsychotics. The most common of these "atypicals" are quetiapine (Seroquel), clozapine (Clozaril), and risperidone (Risperdal).

Possible side effects from atypicals are:

- An increase in the targeted LBD-related behavior,
- The appearance of another LBD-related behavior, and
- Drowsiness.

Although caregivers report that atypicals may cause some LBD-related side effects, such as hallucinations or sleep disorders, they seldom see confusion or increased motor dysfunctions. However, they do see drowsiness. Side effects from atypicals wear off when the drug leaves the body.

> When Anique continued to have hallucinations at home, her doctor prescribed Risperdal. She took it one time and I was up all night because she had such bad dreams. I called her doctor, who prescribed Seroquel instead. It worked and she began to have fewer hallucinations—without the side effects.
>
> —*Jim*

Seroquel is now known to be the atypical least likely to cause serious side effects when used with LBD. In the years since Anique's experience, Risperdal has joined the list of atypicals more likely to cause side effects. Caregivers have also had more negative than positive experiences with aripiprazole (Abilify)[5] and olanzapine (Zyprexa). Clozaril is actually less likely than Seroquel to cause LBD-related side effects, but it can cause serious liver damage even in the general public and must be monitored with regular blood tests. Therefore, it is used only if other drugs are ineffective.

> Emma was having lots of hallucinations, so her doctor put her on Seroquel. Her hallucinations got worse. But Risperdal works fine for her.
>
> —*Howard*

Persons with LBD are different in the way they respond to medications. Emma's experience shows that what works well for most may not be the right drug for your loved one. The doctor may need to try something different, such as the Risperdal that worked for Emma, starting with very small doses and, if there are no side effects, work up gradually to an effective dose. With all such drugs, caregivers say, "Start low and go slow." This is true even for those drugs such as Seroquel that have shown the fewest side effects. You never know when your loved one will be one who responds poorly. Caregivers should also take note of the black box warning that is on all antipsychotics, including the atypicals.

> When we got Emma's prescription, I noticed a black-bordered warning on the bottle saying that there was an increased risk of death for elderly dementia patients. Should she be taking such a dangerous drug?
>
> —*Howard*

The answer to Howard's question is not a straightforward "yes" or "no." The actual wording of the warning is: "WARNING: This medicine is an antipsychotic. It may increase the risk of death when used to treat mental problems caused by dementia in elderly patients. Most of the deaths were linked to heart problems or infection. This medicine is not approved to treat mental problems caused by dementia."[6]

Although it is true that research has shown a small but well-established increase in the risk of death and stroke for older adults with dementia who take antipsychotics,[7] none of the 17 research trials that examined this issue identified LBD patients specifically. Therefore, we do not know whether the danger of death from antipsychotics is actually higher or lower for our loved ones than for people with other types of dementia. What we do know is that:

- Although the FDA has not approved atypical antipsychotics for use with dementia, LBD-savvy physicians continue to prescribe atypical antipsychotics because they still work better than other drugs with fewer side effects.

- Although heart problems and strokes are not generally LBD-related problems, people with LBD are susceptible to infections, and the research has shown that there were more deaths from infections in elderly patients with dementia taking antipsychotics than in those who took placebos.

As you can see, there are reasons for and against using these drugs. Like the balancing act between mobility and cognition, there is also a balancing act with atypicals. You, your loved one, and your doctor need to discuss the dangers thoroughly and balance them with the quality of life that these drugs may provide. Of course, if you choose to use them, do so with great care; use the "start low and go slow" method.

Most caregivers opt for using the drugs. Jim has searched the LBD-caregiver group sites for stories of deaths related to atypicals; he has found none. He did find a great many reports of an increase of the behavior that the drug was supposed to treat, as in Emma's increased hallucinations, or an increase in other LBD-related behavior, as in Anique's bad dreams.

If you opt to use atypicals, your task is to make sure these drugs do the best possible job with the least harm. Monitor their use carefully, watching for side effects, and be sure to keep good records and report changes.

> When using atypicals, be alert for side effects such as an increase in dementia-related symptoms or too much drowsiness. Report any you see to the doctor so that the dosage or time of administration can be adjusted or the drug changed. Also, watch carefully for infections and get them treated quickly.

As the disease progresses, an atypical may become less effective and LBD-related symptoms may reappear or increase. Watch for these changes and report them to the doctor so the medication dose can be increased. Then be alert again for side effects from this increased dose and report any you see.

It is a good idea to keep a record of what medication is given, how much, and when. Then add comments whenever you see something different. This will help the doctor decide what to prescribe.

> Atypical antipsychotics have both useful and possibly dangerous qualities. Caregivers need to discuss the pros and cons of their use with their loved one's physician. If they are used, monitor your loved one carefully for adverse side effects.

Benzodiazepine-Based Drugs

Antianxiety drugs (tranquilizers), sleep aids, and many over-the-counter cold and allergy medications have anticholinergic (dementia-producing) and sedative properties. They are generally considered unsafe for anyone with LBD.

Antianxiety Drugs

Benzodiazepine-based sedatives such as diazepam (Valium), alprazolam (Xanax), clorazepate (Tranxene), and lorazepam (Ativan) have been used for many years to treat anxiety, combativeness, and acting-out behaviors in the general public. A single dose given to someone with LBD can cause heavy sedation or possibly permanent confusion.

Caregivers report that their loved ones can sometimes tolerate small doses of Ativan, the weakest of these drugs. Of course, that is not always the case.

> My Harry's doctor prescribed Ativan for his agitation. It didn't help, and so the doctor increased the dosage. That worked but when my Harry went to sleep, he thrashed about and kept me awake. I told the doctor, who changed the prescription to Seroquel. That finally worked. Harry wasn't so agitated, and he didn't have those bad dreams.
>
> —*Nell*

With the larger dose, Harry's agitation did decrease, but then he started having another LBD symptom—active dreams. Often this is the case with LBD: One problem is fixed but another replaces it.

> *Alternatives:* Doctors may prescribe a very low, carefully monitored dose of one of these drugs—usually Ativan—for a behavior problem like Harry's. However, caregivers report that many of their doctors prefer to start with an atypical antipsychotic such as Seroquel or an antidepressant such as buspirone (BuSpar) or fluoxetine hydrochloride (Prozac).

Sleep Aids

Flurazepam (Dalmane) and temazepam (Restoril) are examples of benzodiazepine-based sedatives used for sleep with the general public. These drugs should not be given to someone with LBD. Zolpidem (Ambien) is a strong sedative with a record of adverse side effects even in the general public, making it a poor choice for someone with LBD.

> *Alternatives:* Trazodone (Desyrel) and divalproex (Depakote) are mild nonbenzodiazepine sedatives often prescribed in small doses for people with LBD. Some doctors also prescribe small doses of a mild antidepressant such as maprotiline (Remeron). An even safer alternative used by some caregivers is melatonin, a natural hormone that regulates sleep.

Quick Review

- Drugs such as Valium, Xanax, and most sleep aids have strong dementia-causing and sedative properties and should be avoided by people with LBD.

- Ativan, a milder member of the benzodiazepine family, is sometimes prescribed in small doses for LBD-related behavior problems.

- Alternative sleep aids include Desyrel, Depakote, and the antidepressant Remeron.

Cold and Allergy Medications

Most drugs in this group are sold OTC, that is, over-the-counter without a prescription. Decongestants such as pseudoephedrine (Sudafed) and antihistamines such as diphenhydramine (Benadryl), loratadine (Claritin), and chlorpheniramine (Chlor-Trimeton) have long been used to treat cold and allergy symptoms. Decongestants and antihistamines usually have some form of benzodiazepine in their active ingredients. Therefore medications with either of these drugs should be avoided. Some drugs, such as antihistamine and nasal decongestant (Actifed) or acetaminophen, brompheniramine, and pseudoephedrine (Dimetapp Cold and Fever) contain **both** decongestants and antihistamines, i.e., **two** dangerous ingredients, making them even more likely to cause problems.

> Just because a drug does not require a prescription does not
> make it safe for someone with LBD. It simply removes the safety
> net of physician and pharmacist and leaves the decision up to
> you. Never give your loved one OTC drugs without checking with
> the doctor or pharmacist first.

All of the drugs in this group can cause LBD-related side effects
such as confusion, active dreams, or hallucinations. Fortunately,
although these reactions may be intense, they are seldom if ever
permanent.

> Hilda has seasonal allergies. She's always had good relief with
> Zyrtec, an antihistamine that's now available over the counter.
> But then she was diagnosed with LBD and started taking
> dementia medications. They really helped. She could think
> more clearly, and she stopped having those active dreams. This
> spring, her allergies came back for the first time in several
> years, so she took one of her old Zyrtec pills. Wow! She was so
> confused—it was like she wasn't taking any dementia meds at
> all. That night the active dreams were back. We stopped the
> Zyrtec of course, and by the next day, she was fine again. We
> tried Claritin, but she had the same results with it. Now what
> do we do?
>
> *—Barney*

Cetirizine, in Zyrtec, and loratadine, in Claritin, are common OTC
allergy and cold medications, and both contain antihistamines. Hilda's
confusion increased when the antihistamines interfered with the effectiveness of her dementia medications. However, her confusion lasted
only as long as the allergy drugs were in her body.

> *Alternatives:* Barney might ask Hilda's doctor about mon-
> telukast (Singulair). Some caregivers report that this nonan-
> tihistamine inhaler had few side effects and worked well
> with their loved one's allergies. However, Singulair is a pre-
> scription drug and therefore expensive in comparison to its
> OTC counterparts.

I read all the labels when I'm getting OTC meds for Emma. I
didn't used to, but once I was in a hurry and grabbed the first

cough syrup I saw. When I gave it to Emma, she got awfully confused and could barely feed herself for about a day. Thankfully, I'd only given her a small dose and by the next day she was all right.

—*Howard*

Howard probably bought a cough syrup containing a decongestant (not all do). For instance, the cough syrup Robitussin is safe to use, but Robitussin DM contains a decongestant. You can check for decongestants by reading the list of active ingredients on the label. If guaifenesin, an expectorant, is the only active ingredient, the medication is probably safe. If there are other active ingredients, such as the decongestants phenylephrine or diphenhydramine, you should consider the drug unsafe for your loved one.

As a rule of thumb, avoid cold and allergy medicines that have initials such as DM, PM, PH, AM, etc., after the brand name. They probably signal the presence of an LBD-dangerous ingredient.

Since my Harry had that bad reaction to Haldol at the hospital, I've made an effort to know more about his medications. The hardest ones for me are the ones I buy [over] the counter for his cough or sore throat. I know I should read the labels, but all those words are so big and hard to understand. I always show what I finally choose to the pharmacist and ask if I've made a good choice. Last time, the lady on duty taught me to find one I know is unsafe and then compare its label to one I'm sure about. If the new medication has similar active ingredients, then I can be pretty sure that it isn't safe for my Harry either. Now that I can do!

—*Nell*

Like Nell, learn to read your labels. Even then, it is a good idea check with either your doctor or a pharmacist—or both—before you give any OTC drugs to your loved one. Start with very small doses and work slowly up to an effective dose. Remember, an effective dose for your loved one may be much smaller than the amount recommended on the package.

> To find out if an over-the-counter drug is unsafe, compare its label with that of a drug you already know is unsafe. If they have similar active ingredients, consider that drug unsafe too.

Antidepressants

Depression is a very common for all people with dementia, and even more so for those with LBD. Fortunately, many depression drugs used by the general public are fairly safe to use with LBD.

Tricyclic Antidepressants

Tricyclic antidepressants such as amitriptyline (Elavil) and methyldopa (Aldomet) are like the benzodiazepines in that they have strong dementia-causing and sedative properties, making them unsafe for anyone with LBD. These drugs have been around for a long time, and you or your loved one may have used them for depression in the past with good success. However, tricyclic antidepressants are seldom used for anyone now because the newer drugs have fewer side effects.

Monoamine Oxidase Inhibitors

Besides being used to treat depression in the general public, monoamine oxidase inhibitors (MAOIs) such as phenelzine (Nardil) are sometimes used to treat the motor symptoms of Parkinson's disease (PD). Like other PD drugs, they have dementia-causing properties and, like other antidepressants, they have strong sedative properties. However, most of all, they can cause sometimes fatal reactions in the general public when used with many other drugs and many foods. Therefore, because the advent of newer antidepressants with fewer side effects, these drugs are seldom prescribed. Like the tricyclic antidepressants, they are a poor choice to use with LBD.

The older antidepressants (tricyclics and MAOIs) are seldom used anymore at all. The newer, milder antidepressants discussed next are also used for anxiety, agitation, and other acting-out behaviors, with few if any negative side effects.

Alternatives: Sertraline (Zoloft) belongs to a family of antidepressants called *selective serotonin reuptake inhibitors* (SSRIs) that have limited sedative and anticholinergic properties.

Caregivers of individuals with LBD have reported few negative side effects with these drugs. The list of SSRIs is very long—some of the most common, besides Zoloft, are fluoxetine hydrochloride (Prozac), paroxetine (Paxil), and escitalopram (Lexapro).

Since David had to quit work, he gets very depressed. We've made it a habit to do regular exercise and all, but he still has times when he's really down. We talked to his doctor and he prescribed Zoloft. I couldn't see any change at first but after about a month I saw a change for the better. Now he even plays with the children sometimes.

—*Maria*

There are a few other miscellaneous antidepressants such as bupropion (Wellbutrin), buspirone (BuSpar), and Remeron, that have comparatively mild sedative and anticholinergic properties. LBD caregivers have reported good results with both of these drugs.

Quick Facts

Antidepressants in the SSRI family and several non–benzodiazapine-based antidepressants are generally considered safe for people with LBD.

Drugs for Controlling Muscle Problems

Muscle Relaxants

Muscle relaxants such as cyclobenzaprine (Flexeril) and carisoprodol (Soma) are used to treat tension headaches, muscle cramps, and constricted muscles. Benzodiazepine-based drugs such as Valium may also be suggested as muscle relaxants. These drugs can all cause dementia-related symptoms such as confusion, hallucinations, and active dreams and therefore are not considered safe for people with Lewy body dementia. The side effects from these drugs, except the benzodiazepines, are seldom permanent.

When Anique was in the hospital and woke up with her muscles contracted, the doctor gave her a muscle relaxant. It did relax her muscles, but she began having hallucinations again.

—*Jim*

As with many of the drugs on the "don't give to people with LBD" list, muscle relaxants often solve one problem only to cause another, sometimes more serious, problem.

> Your loved one's muscle problems may be medication related. The medication record mentioned earlier in this chapter will come in handy when it comes to identifying problems. If you see a pattern of increased muscle cramps or other problems, share your log with the doctor, who can assess the need for dosage adjustments or changes in medications.

Alternatives: Although there are few, if any, drugs that can be recommended to safely treat muscle problems, OTC pain medications such as ibuprofen (Advil) or acetaminophen (Tylenol) may help to reduce muscle pain. However, caregiver-based interventions may be even more effective:

- Decrease the incidents of muscle cramps with:
  - Regular exercise and
  - A calm, quiet, and nonstressful environment.
- Existing muscle cramps may loosen with:
  - Soothing activities such as a massage, drinking warm milk, and even laughing, and
  - Distractions that refocus your loved one's attention onto something else.

Incontinence Drugs

Drugs in this group, such as tolterodine (Detrol) and oxybutynin (Ditropan), are used to stop muscle spasms in the bladder and decrease incontinence. Because incontinence is a given at some point in the LBD journey, it is an issue caregivers must face. However, most incontinence drugs have strong dementia-causing properties.[8]

When Hilda started having problems getting to the bathroom on time, we asked the doctor about Detrol because we'd heard so much about it on TV. Turns out it's a bad one for LBD. Hilda gets confused enough; she sure didn't need something to make her worse. So then we asked if there was anything else. The doc said maybe and maybe not—it depended on if Hilda could tolerate the few that were safer for her—and if they'd do the job. Turns out, the only one she could tolerate didn't help much. So we bought a bunch of Depends.

—Barney

Alternatives: The drug Hilda tried was tamsulosin (Flomax). Other caregivers have reported that it worked well for their loved ones and had few side effects. However, remember that with LBD each person responds differently to any given drug, so it may or may not be safe with your loved one or, as with Hilda, it simply may not work.

> For ways to manage incontinence without drugs, refer to Chapter 5.

Parkinson's Drugs

People with PD will usually take drugs such as carbidopa/levodopa (Sinemet) and benztropine (Cogentin), which tend to relax muscles and make them more functional. However, these drugs fight the action of cognition drugs and provide an ongoing dilemma for PDD families, who must continually choose between mobility and cognition (see Chapter 5).

> Most drugs that treat muscle problems, including incontinence, have strong dementia-causing properties and should be avoided. Tamsulosin (Flomax) may work well for incontinence without causing severe side effects.

Opiates and Strong Pain Medications

Caregivers repeatedly report that their loved ones are overly sensitive to opiates such as morphine and meperidine (Demerol) or other strong pain drugs. A normal dose is likely to cause hallucinations, delusions, and other acting-out behavior. However, the behavior stops when the drugs are out of the system. If a person has PD, this sensitivity can start long before there are any dementia symptoms.

My sister Lucille, who had Parkinson's disease, was hospitalized for cancer treatment and given some strong pain medications. When I visited, she whispered that she had overheard some of the staff in a room across the hall plotting a murder. She was frightened that if they knew she had heard, they would kill her, too. Even after my sister left the hospital and was no longer taking the drugs, she continued to believe her danger was real. Other than that, her thinking abilities seemed about the same and she did not have any more delusions. However, her cancer was growing, and so she went on hospice. When her cancer became painful, the hospice nurse gave her some morphine. Again, she became delusional. This time she was sure the sheriff was there to arrest her. We stopped the medication and the sheriff went away. We tried a half dose and the sheriff was back. Then we tried a quarter dose and, finally, that worked, especially if we gave it to her as soon as she began to hurt.

> Give medication before the pain gets bad. It takes less to keep pain from building than it does to decrease it.

Lucille's delusional reaction to opiates and her positive response to a very small dose are similar to those reported by LBD caregivers. Her sensitivity to these drugs may have been an early symptom of Parkinson's disease with dementia (PDD).

When someone we love is in pain, we want it to stop—the quicker, the better. However, for someone with LBD large doses of strong pain medication may bring other stresses, such as the fear my sister felt because of her delusions. As always, it is the caregiver's job to monitor and report so that the right dosage can be used.

Alternatives: Try the milder OTC pain relievers, such as aspirin, Tylenol, naproxen (Aleve), or Advil, first. If more strength is needed, very small doses of the stronger drugs can often be tolerated.

> Lewy body dementia may cause a person to overreact to pain medication with acting-out behaviors. Very small doses—or, better yet, less dangerous OTC pain relievers—may be effective without the LBD-related side effects.

Inhaled Anesthetics

Inhaled anesthetics, or general anesthesia used for surgery, should be used with extreme care with all elderly people. As a person ages, these drugs become more and more dangerous. This is especially true for people with LBD.[9]

> Right after Peter was diagnosed with mild LBD, we sold our home and moved into an apartment in an independent living facility. Peter had spells of confusion, occasional mild hallucinations, and active dreams, but he was still very functional. We were doing fine and enjoying life. And then Peter fell and broke his hip.
>
> Our doctor warned us about the dangers of surgery for anyone with LBD but Peter was in awful pain, and we decided it was worth the risk. After surgery, Peter was in a wheelchair. I knew I couldn't care for him—I have health problems of my own—and so when he came back from the hospital, he went into the dementia care unit of our facility. I had hoped that the doctor would be wrong, but he wasn't. Peter's confusion quickly increased, along with delusions and hallucinations.
>
> —*Jenny*

Before his fall, Peter's dementia was mild enough that he and Jenny were able to adapt to it and still enjoy life together. For many couples, this can go on for several years with the dementia very gradually getting worse. However, it may be that Peter's case is the more common. After a defining event, such as a serious illness or a surgery, the dementia suddenly increases. Although Peter's doctor had warned them about the dangers of surgery, it was a fairly easy choice. With Peter in severe pain, they opted for surgery. For other individuals, whose need for surgery is less urgent, families may choose not to have it done.

> Anique had constant constipation—a problem she'd had all her life. When her doctor suggested shortening her colon to solve this problem she took him up on it. Anique had been having active dreams for a couple of years before this, but it wasn't until soon after this surgery that she was diagnosed with mild dementia. However, we still coped well and were even able to fly overseas to visit our son. Then, about 2 years after her

surgery, she woke up bleeding. I rushed her to the emergency room. The doctor told me she needed emergency surgery to repair damage from the first surgery. This time, she woke up really confused and didn't get better.

—Jim

Anique had an elective surgery before she had any symptoms that she, Jim, or any of her doctors recognized as dementia. However, if her doctor had been as LBD aware as many are now, he would have asked the right questions and learned about her active dreams, a very early, but also very common, symptom of LBD.

If Anique's doctor had known to warn us about the dangers of surgery for someone with a symptom like active dreams, I think that she would have opted against the surgery. After all, her constipation was annoying, but it hadn't stopped her from living a full life.

—Jim

Not everyone with active dreams goes on to develop dementia. Therefore, it is possible that without the surgery Anique would have been one of those who did not. Alternatively, more likely, rejecting the surgery would have postponed the dementia for awhile, still a worthwhile result. Her second surgery was more urgent and impossible to refuse.

A couple of years ago I had open heart surgery to remove some clogged arteries. Because of my age and my work with LBD, I requested that my surgeon use only those anesthetics that I had read were the safest for elderly people. He laughed. Then he explained that those drugs would not keep me under as deeply or as long as this surgery required. I was basically a healthy man with no LBD precursors, so I opted for the surgery anyway. My risk paid off; I survived the surgery with no cognitive damage and my heart is now working well.

—Jim

Major surgery lasting over a period of hours, as Jim's did, requires strong anesthetics. Like Jim, one may have to evaluate the risks and simply choose for or against the surgery.

My dad has LBD. He required dental surgery awhile back. I'd been a member of an online LBD caregivers support group for a couple of years, and I'd heard the horror stories of loved ones who've had surgery. I didn't want that to happen to Dad, so I did some research. I discovered that with anesthetics like one called propofal, Dad had a much better chance of recovering without additional problems. When I told this to his dentist, she said she'd planned to use these milder drugs anyway. I was so relieved. Because I had checked it out, I didn't worry so much about Dad's surgery. And he did fine; I didn't see any change in his mental abilities.

—Kyla, daughter of Ed

Drugs like the one Kyla mentioned, propofal,[10] are what Jim suggested to his surgeon. These milder anesthetics are often used for dental surgery like Ed's or for minor surgeries that can be done in a short time. The likelihood of LBD-related side effects is much lower with these drugs. Sometimes, there may be other alternatives to general surgery, such as using a spinal injection or a local anesthetic. Any of these may have their own dangers, but they are usually safer than a general anesthetic for all elderly people and especially for persons with dementia or precursors to LBD in their history.

> Surgery with a general (inhaled) anesthetic carries a risk of greatly increased dementia for someone with LBD and the risk of the onset of dementia for persons with precursors of LBD in their medical history.

You, the Expert

Make yourself an expert. Become knowledgeable about drugs that are safe and unsafe, including OTC drugs. Keep careful track of all the drugs your loved one takes and his reactions to them.

Then, speak up. Dare to educate your health care team. Present your information with the understanding that they, like you, are dedicated to providing your loved one the best treatment possible. You will find that in most cases, they will appreciate and use your information. In turn, your health care team can help you to learn more, guide you as you choose over-the-counter drugs, and help you with the drug-related decisions that must continually be made when caring for someone with LBD.

9

Managing Acting-Out Behaviors

Besides the cognitive and movement problems discussed previously, Lewy body dementia (LBD) also causes behavioral symptoms. In turn, these symptoms and other LBD-related dysfunctions, such as poor impulse control, cause various acting-out behaviors (see Chapters 6 and 7). Behavioral symptoms are described more fully in other chapters. However, for the most part, treatment of these symptoms and acting-out behaviors is the same.

Quick Definitions

LBD-related dysfunction: Any symptom that is a part of the Lewy body dementia disorder.

- This includes behavioral symptoms and other dysfunctions, such as poor impulse control, faulty thinking, and depression.

Behavioral symptoms: LBD-related dysfunctions that are in themselves behaviors.

- These include active dreams, hallucinations (perceiving things that are not real), and delusions (believing things that are not real).

- They are often triggered by stress or drug sensitivities.

Acting-out behaviors: Behaviors brought on by an LBD-related dysfunction.

- These include the preceding behavioral symptoms as well as behavior such as angry outbursts, verbal and physical abuse, combativeness, anxiety, agitation,

irritability, clinging, exhibitionism, suspiciousness, paranoia, behavior inappropriate for the situation, inappropriate sexual behavior.

- These are often a person's reaction from an emotional
  level, without a judgment filter.

Medical Treatment

The goal of behavior management is to calm persons with LBD and
bring them to a more acceptable emotional level if not to reality. Drugs
can often do this. The problem is that the drugs that are most effective
with these problems are also those that can be the most dangerous for
persons with LBD.

Quick Review

Drugs used for treating acting-out behaviors include

- *Traditional antipsychotics*
  - Haldol and benzodiazepine-based drugs such as
    Valium have been the treatment of choice for years.
  - Both of these drug families are unsafe for anyone
    with LBD.
  - Very small doses of Ativan (lorazepam), a milder
    drug in the benzodiazepine family, are occasionally
    used successfully along with careful monitoring.
- *Atypical antipsychotics*
  - Seroquel (quetiapine) and similar drugs are often the
    drugs of choice for someone with LBD.
  - These are not always safe and should be used spar-
    ingly and monitored carefully.
- *Antidepressants*
  - Tricyclics and monoamine oxidase inhibitors (MAOIs)
    are not recommended.
  - The newer antidepressants are often milder and safer
    than other drugs.
  - These can be used for acting-out behaviors as well as
    depression.

- *Melatonin*
  - It is a dietary supplement.
  - It is usually safe and can sometimes be effective.
  - Although it is available without a prescription, a doctor should be consulted.
- *Dementia drugs*
  - A person with LBD may already be taking these for cognition.
  - See Chapter 4 for a discussion of action, effectiveness, and dangers.
  - These are comparatively safe and may be all that are needed at the onset of dementia.
  - They lose effectiveness as dementia progresses.

See Chapter 8 for a more thorough discussion of specific drugs for acting-out behaviors, their dangers, and suggested alternatives.

Behavior Management

With all the difficulties that surround drug treatment, nondrug behavior management is an attractive alternative. It should always be tried before drugs are used, and you should continue to use it with your loved one even after drugs become necessary. Often, these techniques work better, and are definitely safer, than drugs. Even when drugs are necessary, good behavior management techniques can decrease the amount of drugs needed. Behavior management skills are something that the family caregiver can learn with only a small amount of training and can incorporate into the daily routine.

Identifying the Reasons

The first step in behavior management is to attempt to identify the reason behind the acting-out behavior. Like good detectives, caregivers must carefully examine the evidence to come up with answers. Consider your loved one's acting out a cry for help. Find and fix the problem, and the acting out will often decrease or even stop.

It is easy to blame the disease for LBD-related behavioral symptoms and acting-out behaviors. Although Lewy body dementia is the initial cause, stress caused by emotional, physical, and environmental issues powers the intensity and frequency of acting-out behaviors as much as, and sometimes more than, the disease. Unlike the disease, over which we have little control, these factors, once recognized, can be changed so that they are less stressful for our loved ones.

Emotional

With the verbal speech difficulties that often appear early in the LBD journey, behavior becomes a major form of communication. With impulse control eroded and a growing inability to reason, communication tends to be all about feelings. If persons with LBD feel good—happy, content, useful, loved, listened to, safe, and so on—they are less likely to act out. When your loved one feels frightened, frustrated, abandoned, useless, or has other negative feelings, his behavior is going to be more disruptive and he is likely to have more behavioral symptoms.

Your loved one's behavior may not match his feeling, and the reason behind that feeling may be irrational, but the feeling is very real. The most obvious emotion is seldom the underlying cause of the disruptive behavior. Feeling that one is invisible may appear as frustration, anger, or agitation, and the feeling of fear may appear as apathy or obsession.

> When Anique became combative, it was easy to see that she was angry. But I couldn't figure out why. Much too late to do any good, I remembered what she said when I told her about bringing in around-the-clock caregivers: "All you want are more women in the house." I had always been the most faithful of husbands but she was feeling threatened—afraid I'd leave her for these other women.
>
> —*Jim*

If Jim had understood at the time that Anique's combativeness was driven by a delusional fear that he would desert her, he might have been able to defuse the behavior with some behavior management techniques. Fear of abandonment is understandably common for someone with dementia. The more dependent on their caregiver a person with LBD becomes, the more frightening the idea of abandonment is. Such fear occurs very often when the decision to place a loved one into a nursing home must be made. Combine this with caregivers' own feelings of guilt at not being able to keep their loved one home, and you have a high-stress situation—a perfect setup for more acting out.

> Common underlying feelings are fear of abandonment, fear of the unknown (change), fear of uselessness, and fear of invisibility (not being heard or understood).

Physical

Physical problems often increase behavioral symptoms. Caregivers soon learn that an increase in behavioral symptoms can signal that something physical may be wrong even before there are any other signs.

Uncle Hank was usually pretty calm, but once in awhile he'd start having active dreams. Once, he even got up in the middle of the night and started stumbling around, ranting about someone breaking into the house. Aunt Dorothy got him back to bed, and the next morning Uncle Hank didn't remember a thing. But Aunt Dorothy remembered that he'd not moved his bowels the day before. She gave him a double helping of prunes and that did the job. No more constipation—or bad dreams.

—Jerry

Urinary tract infections are the physical problem most likely to be causing an increase in behavioral symptoms. However, other infections, or constipation, like Hank had, can do so, too. If you cannot find physical problems, check for hidden injuries.

My Harry kept having more hallucinations than usual, but I couldn't figure out why. We hadn't changed his meds lately, he wasn't having any urinary and bowel problems, there were no obvious stresses, he hadn't watched any violent TV shows, and he seemed healthy enough. And then I noticed he was chewing only on one side of his mouth. I took him to a dentist, and, sure enough, he had a big cavity. He'd been having toothaches! Now that his tooth doesn't ache anymore, my Harry's hallucinations are back to happening just once in awhile.

—Nell

Nell went down her checklist of reasons for why Harry would have increased hallucinations. When none of those fit, she kept looking for some oddity. It might have taken her even longer to notice Harry's one-sided chewing if she had not been looking for a problem.

Environmental

Physical surroundings. With familiar surroundings, where your loved one knows what to expect, he feels safe. However, changes are threatening. Think about what it is like to stand in the dark at the edge of a cliff. You cannot tell how deep the drop is—maybe an inch, maybe a mile. How hard would it be to jump off? How stressful would it be if you were pushed? That is what it is like for your loved one facing change. Therefore, keep stress down by making no unnecessary changes. If change becomes necessary, make it in small increments while maintaining the old environment as much as possible.

Bill Hutchinson had advanced LBD when he and Barbara spent a year in their motor home.[1] They crossed the nation from Alaska to Florida, raising awareness about LBD. Barbara became a master at controlling their environment. Traveling, which involves continual change, is usually quite difficult for a person with LBD. Barbara counteracted this by keeping the inside of their motor home a never-changing environment where Bill could feel safe and comfortable. No matter where they were, Bill had the same easy chair, the same place at their table, and the same bed. When life outside the motor home got too confusing and he started telegraphing his discomfort by acting confused and irritated, the Hutchinsons escaped to their familiar motor home sanctuary. Bill tolerated and even enjoyed the trip.

Barbara also kept the clutter down in their motor home. A too-busy environment, including too much noise, too much furniture, too many people around, too much of almost anything, is another stressor. Remember, choices are difficult for a person with dementia. Therefore, limiting environmental choices, like which chair to sit in or who to listen to, will help to decrease stress and, therefore, acting out.

> I read about the Hutchinsons. Their trip was so unbelievable. I can't imagine taking Mom on such an extended trip, even with a motor home. But I use Barbara's environmental control ideas. I really limit the things in Mom's room. Mom's past the point

where new clothes are exciting—anything new is more likely to be confusing! So even if I get something new for her, I try to make it as like her old things as I can. And I don't keep everything in her room, just one or two dresses in her closet and a few things in her drawers. All of this makes it much easier for Mom to choose what to wear, and that starts her day better.

—Marion, daughter of Clara

Like Marion, most of us would not even consider doing what Barbara and Bill did, but we can learn from them and adapt their ideas to our loved one's needs.

Activities. Variety, which once made activities more fun and challenging, now makes them scary and far too demanding. Formerly easy tasks and hobbies may now be frustrating and difficult, if not impossible. Clara's scrapbooking from the discussion about mental activities in Chapter 4 is a good example.

Mom used to do a page in her scrapbook for each month of the year. She loved to find different ways to showcase all the mementos and photos she'd collected for that month. Then she started doing the same very simple page over and over, with different photos, and now she can't even do that. She can't cut, and she can't put the pictures where she wants them to go, and no way can she write the captions. If I offer to help her, she just shakes her head and starts crying. Then I got out one of her earlier scrapbooks. We both enjoy sitting close together, looking at the pages, and sharing old memories.

—Marion, daughter of Clara

Variety and complexity had become Clara's enemies, and then she lost the ability to do her favorite hobby at all. However, Marion found a way to adapt the scrapbooking into a new, less demanding activity that both she and Clara could enjoy.

Media. People with LBD often perceive what they see on television or hear on the radio as real.

A couple of months ago, Peter was up in his chair, watching a sitcom I'd chosen because I thought it wouldn't be too exciting. Was I ever wrong! I was out in the hall talking to an aide when I heard someone on TV yell, "Duck and dive." And then there was this awful crash—in the room, not on TV. We both dashed into the room. When we found Peter on the floor with his head half under the bed, I knew exactly what had happened. We used to live in Alaska where earthquake drills were mandatory, and everyone learned to "duck and dive" under their desk or something heavy. So when Peter heard "duck and dive" his old earthquake training kicked in. Even though he is so weak it takes two aides to move him from his bed to his chair, he somehow managed to fling himself out his chair and would have succeeded in diving under his bed if his head hadn't hit one of the legs. His head was bleeding, but otherwise he seemed all right. His first words were, "Was anyone else hurt?" He believed the earthquake was real.

—Jenny

Not only does Peter perceive the TV programs he watches as real, but he also often internalizes them and incorporates them into his active dreams. In fact, this was the original reason why Jenny did not want him to watch anything exciting.

Mom was having delusions that she was being stalked, and she was really frightened. I convinced her to change her TV viewing from her favorite cop shows to something less stimulating, and the delusions stopped. Of course, every once in awhile she manages to sneak in a cop show, especially when we have a new aide who doesn't know her, and then Mom has delusions again for awhile.

—Marion, daughter of Clara

TV shows full of violence, action, drama, arguing, or confrontation will often increase behavioral symptoms such as Clara's delusions. When people with LBD cannot discriminate between media and real life, it is up to their caregivers to find ways to monitor their loved one's viewing and eliminate shows that overstimulate or install fear.

Drug Effects

Adverse side effects and sensitivities were thoroughly discussed in Chapter 8, but do not forget to add drug effects to your list of possible reasons for an increase of acting-out behaviors, especially right after a change of medications. Some drugs given for one acting-out behavior may stop the targeted behavior but cause another one. Remember Anique's experience.

The doctor prescribed an atypical antipsychotic to stop Anique's combativeness. She calmed down, but then after she went to sleep, she had active dreams all night long. I called the doctor and he prescribed a different antipsychotic drug and that one worked fine.

—Jim

Alcohol. Although many caregivers report that their doctors tell them that a glass of wine or a can of beer a day can be more soothing than harmful, do remember that alcohol is a sedative, meaning it depresses brain function. Even small amounts can act as an overdose and increase acting-out behaviors. This may be true especially for active dreams. The sedative effects of that evening glass of wine wear off in about 4 hours, and then there is a corresponding stimulant effect that may result in intensified active dreams.[2] Finally, if your loved one is taking any other medication, do not give him alcohol without checking with his doctor first.

David hated to give up his evening glass of wine, but when he did, we found he had fewer active dreams, and the ones he had weren't as violent. I was thinking I'd have to move to another bed, and I'm glad I didn't. I'd miss the closeness we still have at times.

—Marie

The good part is that any side effects from alcohol are temporary. If your loved one really enjoys a glass of wine, and the doctor says it is all right, then allow him to have a small glass an hour or so before bedtime. However, monitor the nights carefully to see if there are more dreams that are active when he has his drink than when he does not.

Quick Review

Things can cause your loved one stress, which can be helped through behavior management techniques, include

- **Feelings that cannot be communicated verbally**. Look for the underlying feeling, and then respond with behavior management techniques.

- **Physical problems**. Fix the physical problem, be it constipation, infection, or hidden injuries, and the acting-out behavior will usually decrease. Look for a urinary tract infection first because it is the most likely cause.

- **Change**. This includes everything from moving to a different house to using a different table setting. Make no unnecessary changes and make those that must be made as minimal as possible—move beloved belongings to the new house, buy the same style of clothes, and so forth.

- **Too much variety and clutter**. Too many choices or too much of anything—furniture, photos, people—can cause problems. Limit choices to no more than two. Limit items and people to only a few at a time. Routines and rituals are less stressful than various activities.

- **Too much intensity**. Things such as loud music, violent TV shows, and arguing can be too intense for a person with LBD. Consider this when choosing activities: play soothing music, monitor TV viewing, and choose less exciting shows, for instance.

- **Too high expectations**. Old hobbies, tasks, and activities may not be possible. Find new, less demanding replacements.

- **Drug reactions and alcohol**. As mentioned in Chapter 8, keep track of the drugs that are unsafe for your loved one and those that can cause unwanted side effects. Be aware that alcohol, especially before bedtime, may cause active dreams or agitation later in the night.

Behavior management techniques are aimed at decreasing the negative feelings that foster your loved one's acting-out behaviors and increasing positive feelings that foster contentment. When persons with LBD are happy, calm, and content, they will exhibit less acting-out behavior, including fewer active dreams, hallucinations, or delusions. Your job will be less stressful, and it will be easier for you to present a calm demeanor—which your loved one will then reflect.

Getting Started

There are a few things you may be able do early on in the disease that can help you and your loved one deal with all of the changes that happen with LBD as it progressively takes away skills and abilities.

Talk About It

Do not make LBD the elephant in the room. For some, this will be easier than for others. Some people want to face their problems head on, and others try to avoid them, hoping that if no one mentions them then they will go away. If you can find a way to discuss what to expect with your loved ones and what their wishes are early on, before dementia has robbed them of the ability to make choices, your job will be easier later. Caregivers repeatedly say that if they have discussed making a change together, persons with LBD are more accepting of the change even if they do not remember the discussion. Include difficult subjects such as the following:

- The things you can do to make the transition easier when driving will no longer be safe
- The things that might make residential care necessary, such as an illness of your own, or anything that would cause an unsafe situation. Also discuss what kind of a residential facility would be acceptable and what features would be the most important to him.
- Financial and legal arrangements that need to be made
- Your loved one's preference in choosing a caregiver in case something happens to you
- Other things that your loved one knows that you need to know—such as where the legal papers are kept

Caregivers suggest that the best way to have this conversation is to make it a discussion about "both of us" and what the other would need to know. This will probably comprise not a single conversation but many short discussions over a period of time.

Write It Down

Once you have answers to your questions, do not expect to remember them under stress. My sister Lucille carefully told me where all of her legal papers were stored: some here, some there, throughout her home. She kept her will, which she knew we would want to see as quickly as possible after her death, in the freezer compartment of her refrigerator. "It's safe there if there's a fire, and no one would think of putting papers in a freezer, so it's also safe from theft," she told me. After the funeral, we wanted to read the will, but I could not remember where she had hidden it. I had not written it down because I was so sure I would remember such a novel hiding place. We had to wait another day to get a copy from her lawyer. I found the will a week later when I cleaned out the freezer.

Stress not only makes things more difficult for someone with dementia; it also makes everyday life more difficult for all of us. Do not depend on being able to remember something later when you may be stressed. Write it down, and keep a running list of everything your loved one tells you that might be important later, even if it is that he likes beets better than carrots.

Also, write other things down. Keep a medical record so that you can show how your loved one is responding to his medications. Keep a daily diary so that, over time, his pattern of fluctuating cognitions can be seen and recognized. Be sure to include not only his thought processes and behaviors but also his motor ability and any physical problems he might be having that day. Because Lewy body dementia is a disease to which no one responds the same, your written record is quite important for your loved one's care.

Join With Your Loved One Against the Disease

People who join against a common cause do better. If right from the start, you and your loved one have agreed that it is "us against Lewy," you will find that being a team will help both of you. When your loved one is acting out, it will be easier for you to see "Lewy" as the culprit. When he wants to do something and cannot, it will be easier for him to be angry with "Lewy" than you. Make it a habit right from the beginning to talk about the disease. Instead of saying, "I notice that you are having more difficulty talking today," you might say, "I see Lewy has your tongue today." Alternatively, during a *good time* you might say, "Lewy's lying low today."

Behavior Management Techniques

These techniques will help you when your loved one begins to have LBD-related symptoms and exhibit acting-out behaviors.

Join Your Loved One in His Reality

Do not try to convince your loved one that what he sees or believes is not real. This *is* his reality, and trying to change it will only cause frustration—for both of you. Instead, accept his reality. Then, without adding to the drama, gently guide him back to reality. The goal is to meet the person where he is, then redirect or distract. Back in Chapter 7, Jim joined in Anique's reality enough to solve the problem when he sent home children coming out from behind the TV. He did not join in the drama by playing with the children.

Barbara Hutchinson tells a story about Bill when he was in a nursing home prior to their LBD drive across America:

> Bill became convinced that one of the nurse's aides was "bad." Usually a very peaceful person, he got combative whenever he saw Nancy and did his best to chase her out of the room. I worked as a charge nurse in a different part of the same facility, and Nancy had been one of my aides. She was a caring woman who would never think of hurting any of her patients. However, I knew it would only make Bill more agitated if I tried to convince him of that, so I asked that a different aide be assigned to him until he "forgot."
>
> —*Barbara*

Bill's behavior toward Nancy was caused by an LBD delusion. Caregivers say that such false beliefs can last for up to 3 weeks but seldom last longer. Barbara's solution gave Bill a chance to forget—to let go of his delusion—because he was not being constantly reminded. Two weeks later, Nancy was reassigned to Bill's section, and he was perfectly friendly to her.

Do Not Take the Behavior Personally

Remind yourself that it is not the person, it is the disease.

> Jake was convinced that I wanted to run away with some other man. He started trying to hit me and became verbally abusive. At first, I was so hurt. I've never given him a reason to distrust me. But then I started telling myself, "It's the disease, not my husband. It's the disease . . . it's the disease . . . it's . . ."
>
> —*Norma*

Jake's delusion is a very common one for someone with dementia. However, that does not make it any easier for Norma to deal with. It is never easy to deal with anger, combativeness, or other acting-out behaviors that appear for no apparent reason. Caregivers say that they have to separate the disease from their loved one daily, sometimes minute by minute.

Respond to Feelings

Identify the underlying emotion behind the behavior. The reason is often irrational, but the feeling itself is very real.

> Jake got so combative that I had to take him to the emergency room. I had just told him we'd put him on the waiting list for a bed in a nearby dementia care facility. It wasn't hard to see that he was afraid I'd put him in there and desert him—just like his son, Harold, had predicted I would. Knowing that fear of abandonment was behind Jake's angry outbursts helped me be less scared.
>
> —*Norma*

Norma had taken a class in behavior management and knew how to look for the feeling behind the anger. Once she figured out that Jake's fear of abandonment was causing his anger, she felt better able to deal with his behavior.

> I waited until he calmed down and had some ability to understand me, and then I got him to talk about years ago when we moved into our first house. As we reminisced about that, I kept emphasizing all along about how much I'd enjoyed having him in my life. We've always been touchy-feely, so I hugged him a lot. He still gets combative at times, but it isn't nearly as bad as it was. I guess he heard me and somehow it stuck.
>
> —*Norma*

Norma did not try to reassure Jake while he was being irrational but waited until he was calmer and could actually hear her. Sometimes, as in Jake's case, this may require using some medication.

People with dementia have a much better handle on the past than they do on the present or future. When trying to reassure your loved one

- Talk about memories from the past that describe what you are trying to convey in the present.
- Support the memories with touch and expressions of affection to show that you still feel the same way.

Stay Positive and Calm, and Do Not Challenge

We all pick up on behaviors first before we pick up on words. People who are losing their ability to reason still react correctly to behaviors and the feelings those behaviors imply. If your behavior is calm and accepting, your loved one will reflect that attitude. Moreover, if you can maintain that calm even in the face of their anger, it helps them calm down, too. However, if you lose your temper, your loved one will become even more agitated and angry. If you challenge them, they will feel attacked and respond with even greater acting out. Such a charged daytime atmosphere also tends to increase behavioral symptoms such as hallucinations and active dreams.

> I've learned to listen calmly to David's tirades, then nod and smile. Usually, he'll calm down, and then I can suggest some distraction, like watching TV.
>
> *—Marie*

Marie has learned not to respond to anger with anger, which would only make the situation worse. Instead, she validates him (nods) and, as soon as possible, distracts him.

To be able to present a calm demeanor, you need to keep your own stress level down—not always an easy task for the 24/7 caregiver. Sometimes you are so busy taking care of your loved one that you forget his caregiver. However, what affects you affects him, so if you are stressed, he will be too, and for him stress equals increased acting out, which in turn will stress you further. Taking care of yourself is the best way to stop this vicious circle. See Chapter 15 for self-care suggestions.

Show Affection and Reassurance

Touching has been shown to be a very effective mode of communication with people who have dementia.[3] Using a gentle voice and giving a hug or a kind touch will go far toward calming your loved one. Norma used touch when she hugged and kissed Jake to show him how much she cared. Marion used touch when she sat close to her mother and shared scrapbooked memories.

Touch and a gentle tone of voice are more important than the words you use. However, persons with LBD may be able to understand what you are saying long after they can communicate with you coherently. Therefore, you do need to make your words caring as well.

Offer Simple Sensory Pleasures

Choose something that you know your loved one really likes. Even in the last days, this can optimize his quality of life.

> Peter has always been a chocoholic. And so when he gets agitated, I offer him a piece of chocolate candy. It will often calm him right down!
>
> —*Jenny*

Other sensory treats might be listening to a favorite song, looking at old photos, or smelling a candle with a favorite aroma.

Distractions

Persons with LBD have a short attention span, and they can usually focus on only one thing at a time. Therefore, distractions can be helpful or harmful. On the helpful side, suggesting a new activity will often distract them from whatever is causing the acting out, but distractions can also prevent good communication. If you want to get your loved one's attention, then decrease distractions.

> Another thing that works when David starts yelling is to offer him something to do. I'll tell him it's time to eat, for instance. He likes to eat, and that seems to calm him down. As long as he is focused on preparing to eat and then on eating, he forgets to be combative. I've also found that if I want to be sure David hears me when he's upset, I have the best success when I'm standing in front of him in a quiet room. Touching helps as well.
>
> —*Marie*

Marie has learned to use distractions well. She offers an activity David finds pleasurable as a distraction from his acting-out behaviors and limits distractions when she wants his attention. Touch is an excellent way to draw your loved one's attention away from other distractions and directly to you.

Keep It Simple

When communicating, use words your loved one understands. Ask questions that have yes or no answers, or those that require a clear choice between no more than two items.

I learned that if I held up two of Aunt Callie's dresses one by one and asked her, "Do you want to wear this one, or this one?" and then gave her plenty of time to process, she could choose which dress she wanted. But if I added a third, she couldn't make up her mind and would start to cry.

—Geraldine

Visual cues help, but do not overtax your loved one with too many choices. Also, be very careful not to ask general questions like "Which dress do you want to wear?" or "What do you want for lunch?"

Keep activities simple by breaking larger tasks into a series of smaller steps. Gently remind your loved one of steps that he forgets, and help with the ones he can no longer do. Again, visual cues like signs or examples help.

Every morning Mom and I brush her teeth. She does the work; I'm along as coach. I tell her how one step at a time, and sometimes I have to show her. I have to remember not to get too far ahead because then I'm giving her too many choices. She gets confused and says, "Oh, dear, I don't know . . . I just don't know . . ." and stops doing anything.

—Marion, daughter of Clara

Working with persons with LBD is like the Alcoholic Anonymous (AA) slogan, "One day at a time," only in this case it is "One step at a time." If you get too far ahead, you lose them.

Use Regular Routines and Rituals

This is another aspect of "keep it simple." Do the same thing every day at the same time, from getting up in the morning to the pre-bed ritual at night. This eliminates difficult and stressful choices. The sameness gives persons with dementia the ability to feel in control—they know what is going to happen next.

Jake sweeps our walkway every day and takes out our garbage after I've bagged it up. When he has regular tasks to do, he's happier and acts out less.

—Norma

Rituals and routines that vary as little as possible and simple but helpful tasks make your loved one's life less stressful. Regular hours for meals, naps, and other activities provide a frame for his day. Helpful tasks, such as those that Jake performs, increase a person's sense of value.

Use the General Dementia-Slowing Measures

Do not forget the general dementia-slowing activities, such as regular exercise, good diet, mental stimulation, and social activity (see Chapter 3). These activities, especially exercise, tend to decrease acting-out behaviors.

> David and I try to go for a mile-long walk every day. We used to go in the evenings, but I noticed that the closer to bedtime we went for our walks, the worse his dreams were. Now we go after lunch. I can tell when we miss a day. That's the night he will usually dream.
>
> —*Marie*

As Marie discovered, it is important to exercise earlier in the day. Exercise near bedtime may be too stimulating and increases the occurrence of dreams.

Learning From Our Children

Dementia is difficult enough for adults to handle; it is especially difficult for the families with children still at home.

> I know that David's dementia is hard on the kids but I'm continually amazed at how well they do with him. They are often better at dealing with his paranoia and irrational anger than I am.
>
> —Marie

Marie and David have two school-age children. Children can be very accepting. They deal with their dad where he is—not where they want him to be. Marie, on the other hand, has a memory of the David she used to know, and it is easy for her to unintentionally put expectations on her husband that he can no longer meet. That is the lesson we can learn from our children: Accept our loved ones where they are. Accept them and give them lots of love and affection. Just that will go a long way toward decreasing acting-out behavior.

Quick Review

- **Talk**. Discuss the disease and your loved one's wants and needs early on.

- **Join together**. Face the disease with your loved one.

- **Accept his reality**. Take part in your loved one's reality enough for redirection.

- **Do not take your loved one's behavior personally**. "It's the disease talking, not my loved one . . ."

- **Respond to the feelings**. When you soothe the feelings, the acting-out behavior decreases. Listen to what your loved one means, not always to what he says.

- **Take care of yourself**. This will help you stay positive and calm.

- **Do not challenge**. When your loved one starts to act out, give him time to calm down.

- **Show affection and reassurance**. Touching, hugging, and generally showing you care is probably every bit as important as listening.

- **Offer simple sensory pleasures**. Increase your loved one's pleasant experiences, and encourage pleasurable activities.

- **Use distractions wisely**. Distractions can be helpful or harmful. Use them to redirect your loved one's attention, and limit them for good conversation.

- **Keep it simple**. Ask questions with no more than two choices. Do tasks one small step at a time.

- **Use routines and rituals**. Give your loved one's life a sense of structure, safety, and usefulness.

- **Use dementia-slowing activities**. Regular exercise can decrease acting-out behaviors.

- **Accept your loved one as he is**. Do not put unreasonable expectations on him.

These few ideas are just some of the basic techniques. If you learn and implement only these, then you will see some good results, but there are many more. Check out the books and articles on behavior management of people with dementia available on the Internet, in bookstores, and at libraries.

Although LBD and AD have some definite differences, coping with the behaviors brought on by dementia is mostly the same, no matter what kind your loved one has. Therefore, check with your local Alzheimer's Association and other dementia-related groups to see if they are offering classes on behavior management. And then, if you possibly can, attend one or more. Nothing helps you learn behavior management like hands-on practice. Other groups may also offer such classes. Jim and I recommend the Beatitudes Campus,[4] a local organization that offers classes to other institutions, groups, and family caregivers nationwide.

We also recommend the Lewy Body Dementia Association, Inc. (LBDA) behavioral issues forum.[5] Here you can learn what to expect, what other caregivers do, what works for them, and what does not. Finally, we recommend two very good articles that you can find on the Internet, one by Ferman, Smith and Melom[6] and another by the Family Caregiver Alliance.[7]

10

Coping With Autonomic Nervous System Dysfunctions

The autonomic nervous system (ANS) is the part of the brain that controls the automatic (autonomous or involuntary) functions, such as temperature regulation, swallowing, blood pressure, digestion, elimination, urination, and sexual functioning. The diagram in Figure 10.1 shows the organs that control these various functions, each of which can be impaired by Lewy body dementia (LBD).

Dementia occurs with LBD when Lewy bodies attack brain cells and decrease the level of the chemical acetylcholine, which is involved in regulating the ANS. This affects the ANS by slowing it down and causing the many organs it controls to function poorly. Therefore, whether it is a temperature control problem, an elimination problem, or anything in between, the initial treatment is often the same.

Most drugs used to treat ANS-related symptoms in the general population are not safe to use with people who have LBD. They may make the problem worse, cause other ANS-related problems, cause dementia symptoms, or increase acting-out behaviors. Therefore, as usual with LBD, caregiver-based interventions become the first line of defense. However, ANS dysfunctions will often respond positively to dementia medications.

The ANS drives many of the systems in our body, and it requires oxygen as fuel. Regular exercise greatly increases the amount of oxygen to the brain and improves the function of even an LBD-damaged autonomic nervous system. In Chapter 3 we provide information about the value of exercise and other ways to slow down dementia. These same techniques improve ANS function.

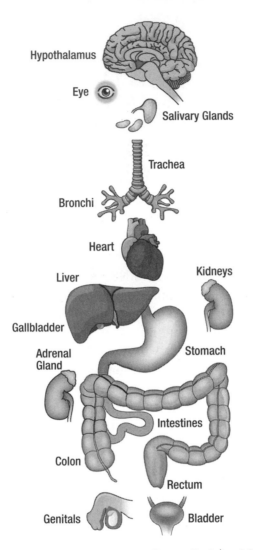

Figure 10.1 The autonomic nervous system affects all of the following organs and related activities.

LBD causes the ANS to slow down. Although you cannot change the effect that LBD has, you can increase the fuel (oxygen) so that your loved one's system can function better, and you can decrease the demand for power. The following suggestions are a good place to start:

- *Exercise:* Increasing the fuel to the brain will help the ANS function better and even be able to handle stress better.

- *Reduce stress:* Stress increases the pressure put on the ANS, and sometimes your loved one's system just bogs down. Usually, it will only get much slower, but sometimes it quits working well at all, and the result is organ dysfunctions, including difficulty swallowing or urinary retention. However, even a damaged ANS functions better with the removal of stress. In Chapter 9 we provide a list of basic stress reduction techniques, and suggestions for stress reduction specific to ANS dysfunctions appear later in this chapter.

- *Use moderation:* When an LBD-damaged ANS is overloaded, it slows down and performs poorly. If your loved one eats too much at one time, for example, the added workload will cause the gastrointestinal (GI) tract to move too slowly to process the food properly. Allowing time between ANS-related tasks such as getting up from a chair and eating will also decrease demands for power.

- *Practice patience:* Because a damaged ANS slows everything down, your loved one needs to do everything, from getting up in the morning, to eating, to moving from one place to another, to toileting, slowly. If you become impatient, it will increase your loved one's stress level, and you will spend more time, not less, on tasks.

- *Add pleasure:* Pleasure decreases stress, but it does more than this; it also adds to your loved one's quality of life. This increases his interest in what is going on, and he will likely be a more willing participant in his own care—and in life in general. It also increases your sense of well-being as a caregiver, which is then telegraphed back to your loved one.

The autonomic nervous system:

- Controls the involuntary functions in the body and
- Works best for our loved ones with:
  - Adequate fuel (oxygen via exercise),
  - A low stress level,
  - Moderation (spread the workload out),
  - Patience (everything takes more time), and
  - Pleasure and enjoyment.

Swallowing

Dysphagia (difficulty swallowing) can start early for the person with LBD. Fluids are the most difficult, but chewing may also become a challenging task.[1]

> Over the last year, Mom's developed problems with swallowing. Sometimes she has so much saliva in her mouth that she drools and gets embarrassed. I worry more about the times when she has such a dry mouth that she has a hard time swallowing.
> —*Marion, daughter of Clara*

Marion's concern over choking is valid.[2] The autonomic nervous system controls sphincters, valves that open and close as needed, throughout the body. Sphincters at the top of the GI tract control the passage of food into the esophagus or the passage of air into the lungs. LBD makes these valves less efficient, and when the wrong valve is opened and liquid or food is aspirated, or drawn into the lungs, infections may follow. Such infections may then develop into pneumonia.

Pneumonia brought about by aspiration is a major cause of death for people with LBD.

Clara takes carbidopa/levodopa (Sinemet) for her Parkinson's symptoms, and dry mouth is one of its side effects. Clara's difficulty swallowing is not only due to her dry mouth. LBD weakens the muscles that facilitate swallowing, so her muscles are also weaker and less efficient than they used to be. For people with Parkinson's disease with dementia (PDD), it is always a balancing act between what these drugs can do *for* them and what the drugs do *to* them.

When your loved one has difficulty swallowing, it is natural for him to limit his fluid intake. Drinking just takes too much effort. Moreover, with aspiration as a common problem, swallowing can be scary as well. Avoiding liquids can lead to dehydration, which is a problem that can be as serious as aspiration, if less dramatic. Without enough fluids in the body, many other ANS dysfunctions can occur, especially urinary retention and constipation, and these are often followed by infections.

Swallowing difficulties may cause poor eating habits and result in malnutrition. Muscles then become even weaker, and your loved one

will feel even more tired. Malnutrition also increases a person's suscep-
tibility to infections and, when infections do develop, they heal more
slowly.

Finally, swallowing difficulties can make eating in public embarrassing. If your loved one cannot eat without coughing, sputtering, and
drooling, he may prefer to eat alone or only with people close to him.
This is just one more way LBD is an isolating disease.

Physical therapy can sometimes help. Certain exercises can
strengthen the chewing and swallowing muscles, and various other
techniques can improve swallowing and decrease choking. Because
your loved one is likely past learning anything new, physical therapy
must be a partnership project, with you learning and directing your
loved one in what to do when—and sometimes even showing him how
over and over again.

Here are some techniques a physical therapist might teach:

- Drinking in a chin-to-chest position.

When I went with Mom to her physical therapy group, the therapist said dysphagia cups would help. I didn't know if it was a
gimmick or not, but I got Mom one anyway. I love it! The cup
makes it easier to do the head-down drinking we learned about,
and she is swallowing so much better now. I used to have to
clean up a mess about once a day because she kept dropping
cups, but this cup has a huge handle and she can get a really
good grip on it. The cup I bought is insulated, and now Mom's
coffee stays hot longer, too.

—*Marion, daughter of Clara*

This chin-down position increases the chances that fluid will go
down the esophagus and into the stomach, where it belongs, instead of
down the trachea and into the lungs, where you definitely do not want
it. The gag reflex is stifled as well. An insulated cup is good for persons
with LBD because it makes their drink more enjoyable for the longer
time that it takes them to drink.

- Have your loved one eat in a sitting or upright position and
  stay upright for 15 to 30 minutes afterward.

Peter is in bed most of the day now, but we try to get him up for
meals. I've noticed that he does a lot better than when we were

just rolling up his bed and he was trying to eat without really being upright. He doesn't choke as much, and I think he actually eats more. Of course, he wants to go back to bed right after he's eaten, but the nurse in his dementia care center wants him to sit up for a half hour after he eats so he can digest his food better. I try to find something to interest him for that time so he won't get agitated. He's come to enjoy it because I save all of my news about our grandkids to tell him then.

—*Jenny*

An upright position helps to keep the sphincter into the lungs closed when your loved one eats. Although a healthy body can digest food in any position, digestion works best when the body is upright. Your loved one's LBD-impaired digestion system needs all the help it can get, thus the added half hour. Sometimes you have to find incentives, as Jenny did, to help your loved ones do what they need to do.

- Avoid foods that are too hot or too cold because these extremes may be unpleasant to anyone with dementia.

Our swallowing therapist told me to avoid extremes. That's when I realized that the spicy Mexican food that Harry had always loved was one of the things he was choking on.

—*Nell*

Too much intense stimuli at once, such as the spicy food, can be as bad as something that is too hot or too cold.

- As the dysphagia increases, you may need to thicken "thin" fluids like water, tea, coffee, milk, and broth.[3]

Even sitting up, Peter was having difficulty drinking. We tried thickening his fluids, and that helped. We started with just a little and kept adding until it was thick enough to help him swallow.

—*Jenny*

People tolerate thickened liquids differently. Before you use thickening at all, try the head-down drinking. Often this is enough for quite awhile, but eventually you will probably need to use some thickening. Use only as much as you need to maintain as much normality as possible, but do not worry about using too much. Even the thicker liquids work to provide your loved one's daily quota of fluid. There are a multitude of commercial thickeners such as Thick-It on the market. You can also use natural thickeners, such as cornstarch or potato flakes.

- Avoid anything that melts or turns to liquid in the mouth, such as ice cream, ice cubes, or juicy fruits such as oranges or watermelon. Also, avoid straws because they can cause choking.

I learned quickly not to give Peter straws. I thought it would make it easier for him to drink, but instead he choked. Peter used to love ice cream, but I've quit giving it to him. The extreme coldness seemed to make him less able to swallow, and then it melted in his mouth and he really had trouble.

—Jenny

Peter might be able to tolerate yogurt as long as it is not frozen. Yogurt can be served at a warmer temperature and is a thicker substance.

- Make dinnertime enjoyable. Provide favorite foods on brightly colored plates that contrast with the food colors.

My Harry was having an awful time getting his food down. Every meal was a battle, with me trying to get him to eat and him choking on nearly on every bite and then refusing to eat at all. Our swallowing therapist had some good suggestions which I tried. First, I took a little time for myself before the meal to relax and calm down. Then I fixed the prettiest plate of food I could, with lots of color and Harry's favorite scalloped pota- toes. I'd been so intent on getting Harry to eat that I hadn't been eating with him. This time, I fixed my own plate and sat with him while we both took our time. When he was resting between bites, I chatted a bit, but I made sure it wasn't anything he had to answer—I didn't want him to get stressed about trying to eat and talk too. It worked. He choked once, but went back to eat- ing. He actually cleaned his plate!

—Nell

Presentation is important but, as Nell learned, a calm and positive attitude is even more important. Because Nell made the meal a time of togetherness instead of a chore, Harry relaxed too. With less stress, his

LBD-damaged muscles worked better, and he was able to get his food down and enjoy it too.

- Avoid distractions. Remember, your loved one has difficulty multitasking, so if his attention is on something else, it will not be on his food.

Harry gets distracted so easily. Anything can catch his eye, a bird flying by the window, something on the floor, or even music, and then he forgets to eat. I've found that I can usually return his attention to eating by saying something matter-of-fact such as "I sure am enjoying these potatoes" or "Do you want a little more meat?" I also moved Harry so he now sits with his back to the window. It took awhile for him to adjust to the new seating, but it sure did improve his ability to keep his attention on his food.

—Nell

Nell has learned to limit her chatter at the table and avoid sounding critical or bossy, both of which would likely increase Harry's stress. Although loud music or music with words is almost always distracting, soft music can often be relaxing. Although change is difficult for someone like Harry, sometimes it is necessary. By keeping everything else the same, Nell was able to change the seating arrangement and cause only a minimal amount distress. Nell learned about what worked for Harry the way caregivers must learn most things about what their loved ones can and cannot tolerate—through trial and error.

- You may need to remind your loved one to chew or swallow.

Sometimes, when my Harry gets too distracted—or just nods off—I have to be very direct and say, "Chew, Harry."

—Nell

If Nell can remain calm, Harry will likely be able to respond and move on. If she sounds frustrated, he is more likely to respond by becoming anxious and may not be able to chew or swallow at all.

- Feed your loved one several small meals a day.
  - Serve about five meals a day instead of two or three.
  - Use small portions and fewer foods for each meal.

The smaller and more frequent portions will be less tiring for your loved one. Equally important, it will also improve digestion.

When I started feeding Jake about five small meals a day, he had less constipation. He likes it, too, because eating is getting a bit difficult. But he's always been a great lover of food and he still looks forward to mealtime.

—Norma

Jake's facial muscles were becoming less functional, making eating a chore. The smaller amounts were not as tiring for him to chew. His LBD-damaged GI tract also functioned better when it had more time to process food and was not being overloaded with too much at one time. Last, but definitely not least, he got a couple more pleasurable events in his day.

Swallowing issues are of concern not only for LBD families but also for anyone coping with dementia, Parkinson's disease (PD), or several other disorders. There are some good articles on the Internet, and one of the best we found is "It's Tough to Swallow: A practical Approach to Nutritional Care of Dysphagia," by Becky Dorner, RD, LD.[4] This article was originally written for residential staff. However, the issues are the same for family caregivers, so it is a good place to start.

Swallowing difficulties:

- Start when the muscles that facilitate swallowing weaken and
- Will be less if your loved one:
  - Drinks with his chin down,
  - Eats in an upright position and stays up for half an hour afterward,
  - Avoids straws,
  - Avoids anything that melts in the mouth, and
  - Eats small meals several times a day.

Once the food has been swallowed, it must be digested in the GI tract, and then the residue must be eliminated. When the ANS is functioning poorly, the whole gastrointestinal tract becomes irregular.

Digestion slows down and sometimes stops, and elimination becomes a problem. LBD caregivers say that too much of their time, energy, and patience are taken up dealing with the results of this irregularity: constipation, fecal incontinence, and diarrhea.

Digestion

Digestion occurs when tiny involuntary movements powered by the ANS cause food to travel through the small bowel from stomach to colon, where the residue (stool) is collected for elimination.

The problems with regularity start because your loved one's LBD-damaged ANS is not providing enough power for the GI tract to move the food along properly. The following are suggestions to improve digestion:

- Encourage exercise and reduce stress.
- Provide several small meals a day.
- Encourage fluids for the GI tract's lubrication, to make everything flow better. See the previous section on swallowing for ideas.
- Encourage a high-fiber diet. Fiber holds the fluids in the GI tract and keeps solids from clumping together so tightly that they cannot be moved easily.
  - Read labels to see how much fiber is in the food. For example, some breads have only 1 g of fiber per slice, others may have three.
  - Good sources of natural fiber are bran, oranges, and kiwis.
  - Use the fruit, not the juice, unless the label states "fiber added."
  - Consider commercial compounds such as psyllium (Metamucil) if you have trouble getting your loved one to eat enough natural fiber.

When the residue at the end of the GI tract is eliminated, you find out how good the digestion process was. If it was good, there will be a soft, well-formed stool. If it was not, the stool will be hard and difficult to expel (constipation) or runny and difficult for your loved one's LBD-damaged anal sphincter to hold back (diarrhea).

Constipation

Constipation occurs when food moves through the GI tract too slowly. Because LBD tends to slow everything down, constipation is more of a problem than is diarrhea.

> My dad was having a lot of trouble with constipation, and when he did have a bowel movement, I usually had to use a plunger because he'd plug up the toilet. Once, it was so plugged that I finally dug the stool out of the toilet, wrapped it in paper towels, took it out to the Dumpster, and threw it in. It clunked when it hit the bottom. Then I knew why Dad complained so much about it hurting when he moved his bowels.
>
> —*Kyla, daughter of Ed*

Ed's large, solid stool was evidence of a poorly functioning digestion system, inadequate fluid, and not enough fiber. Kyla needs to increase Ed's fluids and put more fiber in his diet. If that does not work, she may have to consider some of these caregiver-based interventions:

- Check your loved one's medications with his doctor to see if one of those medications might be the problem. Some, including some of the dementia drugs, draw the fluids out of the colon, leaving very hard stools and causing constipation.[5]

- Prune juice has been used as a natural laxative for centuries. Cooked prunes are even better because they also provide some fiber.

- There are some over-the-counter supplements, such as senna tea and Fruit-Eze, that caregivers have recommended to help with digestion. You can research these on any caregiver site, including the Lewy Body Dementia Association (LBDA) forum.

Finally, if none of these work, you may need to use a mild laxative. Most of the laxatives that are safe for general public are so strong that they are likely to cause diarrhea, which leads to loss of body fluids and potassium. Remember that *strong* is a relative term. Someone with LBD can usually tolerate much less than other people can. Whatever you decide to use, always clear it with the doctor first.

A few laxatives you might try include the following:

- *Polyethylene glycol 3350 (GlycoLax, Miralax):* Many caregivers suggest this OTC laxative.

- *Stool softeners:* These are sold without a prescription. They hold fluid and make elimination easier. Although most stool softeners are safer than actual laxatives, they come in various strengths, so be sure to choose a mild one, such as sennoside (Senokot).

Diarrhea

Diarrhea occurs when the food passes through the bowel so quickly that fluid is not drawn out into the body. It is often accompanied by cramps, evidence of a spastic, or too active, bowel. Because slowness, not speed, is the norm for LBD-damaged GI systems, diarrhea is seldom a problem. However, it may occur:

- Following a bout of severe constipation, as the bowel empties out after being plugged;

- When a laxative is too strong;

- As a side effect to some medications; or

- After eating certain foods. These foods will vary with the individual.

Loperamide (Imodium), an OTC drug of choice for diarrhea, can be used safely with LBD and with the doctor's knowledge, of course. Make sure your loved one drinks plenty of fluids when using Imodium.

Fecal Incontinence

This is an elimination problem, and with LBD the usual cause is a loss of sphincter control. The anal sphincter is a drawstringlike muscle that holds fecal material back until one is ready to pass it out. LBD's debilitating effect on the ANS gradually decreases a person's abilities to control the anal sphincter and, thus, elimination. With cognitive abilities decreasing at the same time that sphincter control becomes difficult, fecal incontinence may eventually move from isolated events to the norm.

We were in the mall when my Harry told me he had to go. I knew from experience that meant that he was going as we spoke. I ushered him quickly to the family bathroom—we only shop in stores with family bathrooms now—and cleaned him up the best I could. But his pants were hopeless; we went home with his shirt flapping around his bare legs. It's funny now but then it was traumatic for both of us.

—*Nell*

Fecal incontinence can also occur with diarrhea, where the stool is thin and being pushed out at an uncontrollable speed. A too strong laxative may turn constipation into diarrhea. Even gentle laxatives may result in fecal incontinence because of the increased urgency they cause.

Mom often has constipation. I can usually tell when she needs a laxative because she gets more confused. We use the gentlest laxatives I can find, but Mom still has accidents. When she was home and still ambulatory, she would try to "clean up" the mess if I didn't stop her. More than once I had to clean up the floor and both walls in the hall—and then put Mom in the shower, clothes and all.

—*Marion, daughter of Clara*

At times like these it can be difficult for caregivers to remember that the patients with dementia are not deliberately trying to "get even" with them. The accidents and the ways your loved one deals with them are not under his control.

The confusion Clara showed, or hallucinations, agitation, or even combativeness, can herald a physical problem such as constipation. If you get rid of the constipation, the acting out will usually decrease. However, as with Clara, even the mildest laxatives can cause their own problems. Few people with LBD can do anything quickly. That includes getting to the bathroom on time, especially with the added urgency that even a mild laxative can cause. Once the accident has happened, Clara was not coherent enough to simply wait and let someone else clean it up. She had to do it "now" and, of course, she no longer knew how, so she made a terrible mess. Most LBD caregivers have their own stories like Marion's. It is one more physical problem made worse by LBD's cognitive dysfunctions.

LBD-safe drugs such as tamsulosin (Flomax) may be prescribed for mild fecal incontinence. These drugs relax the bowel and allow for better sphincter control. Adequate fluids and the prevention of constipation will also help. However, as the disease progresses and your loved one's ability to control his anal sphincter decreases, these drugs may not be enough. Fecal incontinence may become as much a fact of life as urinary incontinence.

Here are some caregiver ideas:

- Developing a toileting regimen that matches those times when your loved one has usually had bowel movements in the past may help eliminate fecal incontinence. Remember that people with dementia do well with regular routines. Be careful to maintain a routine once you start.

- Adult diapers and Depends may help contain the problem; however, they are not an all-day answer. You need to take the covering off as soon after a bowel movement as possible and clean the area to avoid infections from fecal contamination.

- Maintaining good general hygiene helps avoid the spread of infections from fecal material in general or from infectious diarrhea.

- If constipation persists, enemas may be necessary. Enemas should not be used unless all other efforts have been tried and should be discussed with the physician first.

You can usually work out a good system for toileting at home. It is not quite so easy when you are out shopping, so it pays to do some research first and find out where the bathrooms are and whether there is a family bathroom. Dealing with bathroom issues in a public place is challenging enough without having to ask where the bathroom is or deal with the stares of people of the opposite sex while you toilet your loved one. Family bathrooms are a wonderful answer to that last issue and worth "scoping out" ahead of time so you will know which stores to frequent.

> Make your shopping and outings easier. Know where the bathrooms are in the stores you frequent. If you can, only frequent stores with family bathrooms.

For more ways to assist your loved one with this exhausting problem, visit the LBDA constipation forum.[6] You will find information about various elimination problems, along with many suggestions and resources. If all you want to do is read, you do not need to join. However, if you want to comment you will have to sign up.

Temperature Regulation

People with LBD may feel hot, then cold, for no discernable reason. However, being cold is more common. Caregivers often report that their loved one is always cold, sometimes when the temperatures are in the 80s.

Layers of clothing works best for temperature control, so keep clothing like sweaters and lap robes handy. You want to make sure that each garment is easy to don and remove. Cardigans are easier than pullovers or sweatshirts, for instance.

> I swear my Harry's internal thermostat is worse than mine was during menopause! He's hot and then he's cold and then he's hot again. He was really struggling with his sweater until I found one with raglan sleeves. The bigger armholes made it easier for him to put it on. He's cold more often than hot, so I was covering him in his wheelchair with a doubled-over blanket. It kept him warm but it was awfully heavy and cumbersome for him to handle, especially if he wanted to drag it back on after he'd thrown it off during a "hot flash." Then I found this lap robe. It's warm enough and he can manipulate it better. My Harry's always been partial to Irish Setters, so when I picked out the one with photos of these dogs all over it he was really happy. He sits, covered up with his lap robe, and pets his "doggies" and grins.
>
> —Nell

As Nell found, smaller lap robes are easier than blankets to manipulate. Her idea of finding a sweater with wide sleeves helped too. Always try to add pleasure where you can, as Nell did with the Irish Setters.

Blood Pressure

Orthostatic hypotension (OH), or low blood pressure upon rising, occurs in about 50% of people with LBD but only 5% of those with just PD. When anyone rises from a horizontal position, blood naturally pools in the lower extremities, decreasing the volume of blood available for the heart to pump, which lowers the blood pressure and the amount of blood pumped to the brain. Normally, the ANS immediately constricts the body's blood vessels and the blood pressure returns to normal so quickly that you do not even notice a problem.

Anyone who has had a surgery has probably experienced OH. Surgery, especially with inhaled anesthetics, is hard on anyone's ANS. It takes awhile for even a healthy body to adjust after this assault. If you have ever had surgery, you may have felt dizzy when you first sat up. That was orthostatic hypotension. The nurse probably would not let you stand until the dizziness passed, either. The dizziness was your warning that your blood pressure was so low that your brain was not getting enough oxygen to function properly. If you had tried to walk too soon, your brain might have had a "power failure" from lack of fuel—oxygen—and you would have fainted. Of course, in a short time you were probably back to normal and could get right out of bed and walk away with no dizziness.

> When Anique woke up in the mornings, she'd be really dizzy. We learned that she needed to sit on the side of the bed for awhile before she stood up. If she got right up from bed, she'd take a few steps and just crumple to the floor in a faint. Then, if she just sat there on the floor for a while, she was able to get up and do fine.
>
> —*Jim*

What Anique was experiencing was similar to what you may have experienced temporarily after surgery. However, her OH was caused not by a temporary stress but by an LBD-damaged ANS. It did not go away, and it was waiting to happen every time she rose from a horizontal position, or sometimes even from a chair.[7] Sitting on the edge of the bed—or the floor, if she collapsed—gave her sluggish system a chance to get enough blood to her brain so that she could stand without being dizzy. People with OH must get up in steps: first sit up, then rest until the dizziness stops, and finally stand up.

Orthostatic hypotension can be lethal. If the slowness is extreme, the body may be unable to adjust in time to keep the heart beating. This is called *syncope*, which starts out with dizziness and fainting, then it was suggested to change to a coma, and can end in death. Fortunately syncope is unusual. The greatest danger of OH lies in the falls and injuries that occur when a dizzy and unstable person attempts to move around unaided.

> • Orthostatic hypotension (low pressure upon rising) causes dizziness and fainting, and in extreme cases death, but its biggest dangers are injuries from falls.
>
> • Use a pressure alarm pad, placed under your loved one, to warn you that he is trying to get up from bed or chair without help.

Treatment

Your doctor has the choice of several drugs to treat orthostatic hypotension:

- *Midodrine (ProAmatine):* This drug lowers blood pressure by constricting blood vessels continually, without respect to need, while it is in the bloodstream.
- *Pyridostigmine (Mestinon)*[8]*:* The action of this medicine works only when the blood pressure is too low. Thus, Mestinon works best with OH, although occasionally ProAmatine may be added for increased effectiveness.
- *Fludrocortisone (Florinef)*[9]*:* A corticosteroid, Florinef is sometimes used to raise blood pressure and can be used safely with LBD. Although its action is different from ProAmatine and Mestinon, it also raises blood pressure without respect to need.

Although Mestinon appears to be the best drug for someone with LBD, remember that everyone with this disease responds differently to drugs. Your doctor may need to try several drugs or combinations of drugs before you find one that works well. The good news is that these drugs can all be used safely with LBD.

Orthostatic hypotension can often be controlled without medications or with less medication if the caregiver is alert for the problem and follows some of these suggestions[10]:

- Have your loved one sit on the side of the bed for at least 10 minutes before standing to give his body time to adjust.

I always have Jake sit on the side of the bed for a few minutes until he stops being dizzy. Awhile back, I helped him sit up and told him to stay there while I got his robe. As soon as my back was turned he stood up and tried to walk. I hate to think what would have happened if I hadn't been close enough to catch him before he fell!

—Norma

This is one of the many instances where LBD hits twice: once as a physical disability (the OH) and again as the lack of cognitive skills needed to deal with the disability safely. Norma learned the hard way that Jake needed constant supervision while he waited. Jake's getting up too soon was not a matter of being obstinate or acting out. With a decreased ability to relate to cause and effect and little impulse control, Jake simply did not understand "You have to sit here until you can stand without falling."

- Include adequate sodium in your loved one's diet. Salt increases blood pressure. With a higher starting blood pressure, OH may not be as troublesome. Your doctor may even prescribe salt tablets to ensure that your loved one is getting enough sodium.

- Avoid prolonged bed rest. When the body lies prone, the blood spreads evenly throughout the body. The longer your loved one spends in bed, the more the blood spreads out, and the more difficult it is for a damaged ANS to get adequate blood to the brain when he stands up.

- Elevate the head of the bed about 4 in. This decreases the amount of work the ANS has to do to get the blood pressure back to normal when your loved one sits up.

- Have your loved one wear compression stockings. This keeps more blood in the upper body, closer to the heart.

Sexual Dysfunctions

Sexual dysfunctions are uncommon for women with LBD, or at least they are seldom mentioned by the literature or by caregivers. Erectile dysfunction (ED) is the most common sexual dysfunction for men with LBD. This may be one more ANS problem, or it simply may be caused by dementia in general. In either case, the result can be low self-esteem, especially for the man in the early stages of LBD. Impotence itself is quite common with any with dementia, especially in later stages. On the other hand, sometimes there is an increased libido, causing inappropriate demands for sex, or forgetfulness, leading to excessive demands for sex. Any of these sexual dysfunctions can reduce personal contact, such as hugging and general touching, which has many emotional consequences. Eventually, most people with dementia will lose any interest in sex. However, their insecurities may remain.[11]

> About the same time my Harry was diagnosed with LBD, he became impotent. I told him it didn't matter, that our love was based on much more than sex. At the time, he seemed to accept that. But then he started accusing me of infidelity. We've had such a wonderful time together that I couldn't possibly think of another man in that way, and until Lewy hit, my Harry knew this and felt the same way. But now every time I leave for even a short time, he assaults me with accusations when I come home. It was bad enough when he was just yelling at me, but now he's trying to hit me. My Harry was always such a sweet man. I can't believe he's doing this!
>
> —*Nell*

It is possible that a change of medications will stop Harry's delusions. However, fears that one's spouse will leave for another person are very common with LBD, especially if there are any sexual dysfunctions, such as Harry's impotence. However, it can happen with women as well.

> After my wife Anique's surgery, she became too difficult for me to handle by myself. I had a caregiver coming in for several hours a day, but Anique needed around-the-clock care. When I told her I was hiring another caregiver, she became very angry. She told me, "You just want more women in the house." I tried to explain that I really needed help, but she just wouldn't listen.
>
> —*Jim*

As Jim's present wife, I can attest that he is the most faithful of husbands, and I am sure that Jim was equally faithful to Anique. However, as her condition degenerated all she could comprehend was how unattractive she felt. She projected that feeling onto Jim and "knew" he did not want her anymore.

I know now that you can't reason with someone with dementia, anymore than you can reason with a drunk, but I didn't know that then. What I did learn was that when I tried, it made her even more angry.

—*Jim*

Jim's efforts to reason with Anique probably made her feel even less heard, less wanted—and more angry. If Jim had known some of the behavior management techniques discussed in Chapter 9, he might have been more successful.

Sometimes, a person with sexual insecurities acts these out in a more aggressive fashion.

David has become a sex maniac. He wants to have sex with me all the time, and he's really inappropriate. Last night we had company, and out of the blue, he said, "Hey, Marie, I'm horny. Let's go to bed," just as if our friends weren't there. I was so embarrassed. They soon left, but I have to tell you, I was in no mood to make love. I was steaming. I knew it was Lewy talking. David was always a considerate lover and would never have embarrassed me that way before Lewy, and that made me feel guilty so I gave in. But the anger was still there, and I knew he could tell. Then I felt even guiltier.

—*Marie*

David's aggression is another way that people with LBD can act out sexually. Without any impulse control or ability to judge cause and effect, they do not perceive that their behavior is getting just the opposite result that they want from their partner. Once, Jim and I went to visit our friend Lilly and her husband, Marvin, who has LBD. We had been there only a few moments when Marvin asked, "When are they leaving?" It was plain to all of us that Marvin was feeling overwhelmed and wanted the security of his wife's full attention. David was likely having similar feelings. In his mind, what better way to get Marie's undivided attention than to take her to bed?

Jim believes that caregiver "turnoff" is the most common sexual problem for LBD couples. Behavior like Harry's paranoia, Anique's accusations, and David's inappropriate demands may replace prior qualities of warmth, caring, humor, or playfulness and make one's once-enjoyable partner much less sexually attractive. Poor hygiene or a request for sex soon after a marathon of cleaning up an unpleasant and smelly accident may make the act distasteful to a normally caring spouse.

Treatment

Drugs such as sildenafil (Viagra), tadalafil (Cialis), and vardenafil (Levitra) are available for erectile dysfunction and appear to be safe to use with LBD. These may be especially helpful for the younger person with early onset dementia. However, most caregivers report little need for medical intervention. Please check with your physician before using any erectile dysfunction drugs.

Sexual issues are very personal, and each couple has to find their own solutions. However there are some guidelines:

- When your loved one is inappropriate, remember how it was, not how it is with LBD. "It's Lewy talking. It's Lewy talking. It's Lewy . . ." This may help you let go of your anger at the Lewy-driven inappropriateness and make you able to respond lovingly.

- Substitute sexual enjoyment that does not include intercourse when that is no longer possible. This will serve to decrease insecurities and will be good for the relationship. Remember, life goes on, even with LBD, and the more normal you can make it, the better both of you will feel.

- Include affectionate hugging, kissing, and touching in your daily routine even after any urge for sex has stopped. Intentional touching for the purpose of showing love and caring is different from the touching that occurs for "business purposes," such as during a transfer from bed to chair.

The bottom line is that dementia does not decrease a person's need to give and receive expressions of love. However the form of these expressions changes as the disease progresses.

11

Coping With Urinary Tract Dysfunctions

Every Lewy body dementia (LBD) family can expect to deal with urinary dysfunctions on a daily basis. Many are due to the weakening of the autonomic nervous system (ANS). However there are also some other urinary problems common with LBD.

Incontinence

Urinary incontinence, the inability to control one's urinary sphincter, is universal in almost all dementias. Controlling one's bladder is a learned response, and as your loved one forgets what he has learned, eventually this goes too. And for a person with LBD there is more than just forgetting. His LBD-damaged ANS is in charge of sphincter control, and gradually this muscle weakens and becomes unable to do its job, often even before your loved one has forgotten how, causing him stress and embarrassment that someone whose dementia is further developed may not feel.

With incontinence, infections or pressure sores develop much more easily, especially if the area is not kept clean.

> Peter's been incontinent since he came out of the hospital with his broken hip. I'm so thankful to the aides here. They keep him cleaned up and try to keep him from developing any skin infections.
>
> —*Jenny*

Because LBD is an illness of the elderly, many caregivers are also elderly persons and may have illnesses of their own as well. Jenny was not capable anymore of the cleaning-up chores her husband required.

This is when either assistance in the home or entry into a residential facility becomes imperative. Otherwise, infections are a continual risk, and with infections come acting out and, worse yet, a general physical decline.

Believe it or not, dehydration can also cause incontinence.

> Anique sometimes became so dehydrated that I had to take her to the emergency room to get a "hydration boost." They'd put in an IV and infuse her with fluids. She'd be good to go for awhile, until it happened again. The problem was that she was incontinent. "If I drink more it will just all come out, and I can't stop it," she told me. And so I just couldn't get her to drink.
>
> —*Jim*

Limiting the amount that comes in to decrease the amount going out does seem to make sense. However, it does not work quite that way. A certain amount of fluids is actually necessary for the bladder sphincter to work properly. Thus, Anique's refusal to drink made her more susceptible to incontinence, not less. This "more fluid will cause less incontinence" explanation can be quite confusing to a person with a limited ability to take in and process new information.

> Dehydration causes a buildup of irritating salts in the bladder, decreasing sphincter control.

At the time, Jim did not know this himself, so he could not have explained it to Anique. He did not even know the questions to ask, let alone the answers. That is frequently the case. All of a sudden, a caregiver is thrust into a situation that requires her to perform a task for which she is unprepared. The good news is that there is much more information available for LBD caregivers than there was a few years ago.

For persons in the early to middle stages of LBD, incontinence can be so embarrassing that they are unwilling to leave home. The isolation this brings about is a major issue with dementia and increases as the dementia progresses.

> Mom quit going to church when she became incontinent. I tried to get her to use Depends and go anyway, but she was too embarrassed. I'm glad they have church services in the dementia care center because she's going again now.
>
> —*Marion, daughter of Clara*

With LBD, urinary incontinence can start even before impulse controls are seriously damaged. Clara, with her inhibitions still intact, felt embarrassed, and this increased her isolation. Being able to control one's bladder is one of the first hallmarks of "growing up," and finding oneself unable to control it as an adult often causes feelings of loss.

In Clara's case, her move to the dementia care center meant that her isolation was reduced, which is a great advantage. In residential centers there is a "we're all in this together" mentality that reduces the isolation caused by problems such as incontinence. However, family still needs to be heavily involved to prevent feelings of abandonment.

Treatment

There are some medications that can be used for bladder control, although the drugs of choice for the general population are discouraged for people with LBD.

- *Oxybutynin (Dridase or Ditropan), tolterodine (Detrol LA), and solifenacin (Vesicare):* These drugs can increase dementia symptoms and should *not* be given to someone with LBD. (Some caregivers have reported success with Vesicare, but it should be used only with a physician's direction and careful monitoring.)

- *Terazosin (Hytrin):* Although Hytrin does not increase dementia, it lowers blood pressure, making it another poor choice for someone with LBD.

- *Tamsulosin (Flomax) and finasteride (Proscar):* These two drugs are usually safe for use with LBD, but they may not be effective, especially late in the disease.

The best bladder control is often attained by the caregiver. Here are a few of the many suggestions Jim has compiled:

- Stop water intake 2 hours before bedtime to decrease nighttime incontinence. This works only if you make sure your loved one gets *adequate fluids* in the daytime.

- Scheduled toileting regimens may help, even if your loved one's dementia is more advanced. Have him void every 2 hours, whether he feels a need to go or not. Regimens, once started, can indicate security to people with dementia, and so they often adapt well to them—and miss them if you should lapse.

• Simplify clothing to make toileting easier.

Jake wears sweat pants all the time now. They are easy to pull down and up, and sometimes he doesn't even need my help. When I do have to help, it's easier for me too. We've had fewer accidents since I got rid of his beloved jeans. In fact, he was so happy with his new "freedom" that he didn't miss the jeans.

—Norma

Loose clothes with elastic or hook-and-loop fasteners (Velcro) instead of snaps, buttons, zippers, or ties make dressing and undressing much easier, or often simply possible. Use adult diapers, especially when going out of the home.

Mom hated her diapers at first. "They make me feel like a baby," she told me. But I noticed that after I convinced her to try them, she was more willing to wear them, especially when we went out. Now I can take her out once in awhile and not worry about accidents that I can't handle.

—Marion, daughter of Clara

Like Clara, once persons with LBD are used to diapers, they will likely be more willing to go out in public because they know they will not have an embarrassing accident. The adult diapers on the market now stop most of the smell and are very absorbent.

> If your loved one suddenly becomes more incontinent than normal, check for physical problems such as an infection or hidden injury. Some people become incontinent when other things are wrong, just as some develop behavior problems.

Urinary Retention

When your loved one cannot empty his bladder despite the urge to do so, it is called *urinary retention*. It occurs when the damaged ANS slows the passage of fluids from the kidneys to the bladder and is common for more than one third of people with LBD.[1]

However, dehydration due to inadequate fluids can also cause urinary retention, even in people with a healthy ANS. Anique refused to drink to avoid incontinence. Other persons with LBD refuse to drink because they know it will lead to a trip to the bathroom and getting from wheelchair to toilet and back again is just too tiring. Some refuse to drink because of an often valid fear of choking when swallowing, whereas others simply quit drinking before they have had enough to hydrate their system because drinking takes too much effort.

Treatment

As is the case for most ANS dysfunctions, drug treatments for urinary retention are limited. Although bethanechol (Duvoid or Urecholine) is used for the general population, it may increase motor dysfunctions and should not be used with any Lewy body disease.

Catheterization, in which a tube is threaded up the urinary passage (urethra) into the bladder, may be needed if retention becomes painful. This may be a one-time or a regular event. In some cases, a full-time catheter, with a clip on the tube to keep it from draining all the time, may be needed. Such a catheter must be inserted by a medical professional and should be chosen only after all other possible solutions have been explored. As with any invasive procedure, there is always an increased risk of infection.

The responsibility for maintaining adequate hydration and preventing urinary retention falls mostly to the caregiver. Here are some suggestions from other caregivers:

- Maintain good preventative care, especially adequate fluids and exercise.

- Good personal hygiene helps maintain an open urinary tract. Any time the urine cannot run freely when the urinary sphincter is released, the fluid will back up and can cause a urinary infection. Be especially careful to avoid getting fecal material in the urinary tract because it can plug up the tract, which greatly increases the chances of infection.

- Sometimes, the sound of running water stimulates the urge to void. Try running water in a sink, shower, or bathtub while your loved one is trying to void. If that does not work, try sitting him in a warm bath or under a warm shower if bathing is not possible.

- Some foods may help keep the urinary tract open. Caregivers have suggested bananas, parsley, or honey. They also recommend avoiding spicy foods. Remember that persons with LBD have a very individualized ability to digest and assimilate foods just as they do with drugs. Each person will react differently to different foods. The best solution is to experiment and see what happens.

Urinary Tract Infection

A urinary tract infection (UTI) is usually a secondary symptom resulting from urinary retention, poor personal hygiene, or both. As the disease progresses, UTIs become an unpleasant fact of life for patients with LBD and their caregivers, and it can be difficult to identify a specific cause. Left untreated, UTIs increase acting-out behaviors and can become major health problems.

> UTI symptoms include pain and burning upon urination, a need to urinate repeatedly without much success, and blood in the urine, as well as nausea and vomiting.

Sometimes, there are no symptoms of a UTI at all. And sometimes an LBD-fogged person is not able to recognize or communicate the symptoms that are there. In that case, you may see an increase in acting out, hallucinations, or agitation—the body's cry for help.

Jake is beginning to have difficulty swallowing. Our health aide and I are continually trying to get more fluids down him. Sometimes, he just gets too tired and pushes the cup away and won't drink anymore. Last week, Jake was awfully weak and he was having way more hallucinations than usual. I knew he was getting dehydrated, so I called the paramedics. They took him to the ER and gave him IV fluids and did tests to see if he had a UTI. I wasn't surprised when the tests showed he did—that's why he was having so many hallucinations.

—*Norma*

The preceding scenario is played out often in LBD families. Limited fluid intake leads to dehydration and urinary retention. Together, these bring on a urinary tract infection; the person with LBD acts out in some way in reaction to the discomfort. The caregivers call for help and their charges ends up in the emergency room, where they get rehydrated, put on antibiotics, and sent home.

Treatment

A UTI is one of the few LBD-related illnesses that can be treated the same as it is treated for any elderly person. However, it is also one that must be treated professionally. Caregivers should not try to treat it themselves. As soon as you suspect a UTI, take your loved one to a doctor to be tested. If an infection is present, the doctor will prescribe antibiotics. Make sure that the whole prescription is consumed. Using the medication only until a person feels better may result in a resistance to that drug that will make it ineffective the next time it is used.

Prevention is the first line of defense for urinary tract infections, and, of course, this job falls to the caregiver. Here are some suggestions:

- All of the earlier suggestions for preventing dehydration and urinary retention apply, along with those for keeping the area clean.

- A daily glass of cranberry juice may help keep the urinary tract open.

I give my Harry a glass of cranberry juice every day, and I drink one too. My granddaughter got us started. She was having problems with reoccurring urinary tract infections after her baby was born, and her doctor told her to drink cranberry juice. It worked for her and when I told her my Harry was going from one UTI to the next, she told me to try it. I can't say it's stopped the UTIs altogether, but he sure doesn't have as many. And I haven't had any. Well, of course I didn't before either, but I like the taste. I put the pretty red cranberry juice in wine glasses and make a party of it. We have a toast and then we drink it down together.

—Nell

Cranberry juice may have a slight resistance to bacteria, which could lessen the reoccurrence of UTIs.[2] Cranberry juice is useful as a deterrent, not as a cure. Once an infection is present, it must be managed medically. Cranberry juice is not just for the elderly. Many women, like Nell and her granddaughter, drink it every day as a preventive measure.

Again, Nell added fun to her caregiving tasks when she made drinking the cranberry juice into a daily toast.

> As the disease progresses, it may become almost impossible to prevent urinary tract infections. It then becomes the caregiver's job to identify them quickly and get them treated.

Although urinary problems can cause many inconveniences, one can still live a full life around them. This is especially true if you adapt by using adult diapers as appropriate and get the frequent UTIs treated quickly.

12

How Do I Build a Health Care Team?

Being a caregiver of someone with Lewy body dementia (LBD) is like being a companion, a nurse, a psychologist, a teacher, and a social worker all rolled into one. We have already addressed the nursing, psychological, and some of the teaching aspects of being a caregiver. The next three chapters are about being your own private social worker.

A social worker is someone who helps people find health care–related resources and supportive services. As your loved one's disease advances, he will need various professionals and services, and it will likely be up to you to secure them. In addition, caregivers must deal with financial, legal, and social issues.

Like nurses, social workers are also teachers. The caregiver of someone with LBD will find herself teaching about the disease everywhere she goes—at home to her family and the health care aide, at the store when she buys supplies, at the doctor's office when she finds that she knows more about how LBD affects her loved one than the doctor does, and so on.

Educating Yourself

Your first task is to educate yourself. You have already started by reading this book. The easiest way to learn more is to use the Internet, because the information is so readily available there. Go first to the Lewy Body Dementia Association (LBDA) Web site (www.lbda.org) and look at the resources offered there—articles about all aspects of LBD, records of ongoing clinical studies, books for sale, and much more. Study the LBDA brochure, which you can get free from the Web site, and go to the LBDA forums and read some of the entries there.

Even better, sign up and become a forum member so you can ask questions and share your own story. Find out how to access online support groups, and look for any local support groups in your area.

Once you have digested what the LBDA has to offer, you can go to some of the resource sites recommended in this chapter and in the resources section at the back of the book. If you want to go further, check out the articles in this book's list of references. Finally, you can simply type "Lewy body dementia" and whatever symptom you are interested in at the moment, such as "swallowing," into Google or another search engine.

> If you do not have a computer, your local library should have some available for use, often free of charge. If you know someone with a computer, ask for assistance. Start by asking your helper to download an LBDA brochure and in the Online Resources section in the back of this book. These will give you a good foundation of knowledge.

Take your time—do not try to learn everything at once. The best thing to do is to read something and then discuss it with someone else—a friend, a relative, or even your home health aide. If your loved one is in a facility, talk to the staff there. Use the information you learn to try new things and then share your experiences. Learn by reading, then sharing, then doing, then sharing again.

This is where a good support group comes in. Support group members are great for sharing information back and forth. You can find out about support groups in your area by checking with the LBDA or the basic resources in the section that follows and at the back of the book.

Some Basic Resources

The following is a list of some good general online references that offer help for finding local services such as health care agencies, residential facilities, and even physicians. Although none of these sites specifically caters to the LBD caregiver, they are still gold mines of information. For example, many articles have checklists and guidelines for choosing various services. These checklists are general, so you will want to add some LBD-specific items. Again, go slowly, read a little at a time, and do not get overwhelmed by all the information.

If you do not use a computer, ask your computer helper to help you research these sites and print copies of the information you need the most. If possible, sit with your helper when the sites are accessed so you can decide on the information you want printed. This may take more than one sitting. Because you need different services, you may want to review these sites repeatedly.

ElderCare Online's Neighborhood Network[1]: When searching for senior services available in your state, this site is very helpful. The home page for this service, ElderCare Online,[2] also offers various other valuable caregiver information.

Family Caregiver Alliance[3]: This is another site that allows you to search for senior services by state. It also includes various excellent information on caregiving.

National Association of Area Agencies on Aging[4]: This site has an Eldercare Locator for local services such as financial or legal assistance, caregiver programs, aging and disability resource centers, and adult day care. You can also call 1-800-677-1116.

Full Circle of Care[5]: Here you can search for senior services specific to home and residential care, hospice care, legal assistance, your local ombudsman, and much more.

Medicare[6]: This government site allows you to compare hospitals, home health agencies, and nursing homes as well as Medicare-related health plans in your area. You can also find physicians and neurologists who will accept Medicare and suppliers of medical equipment in your areas.

See Online Resources (Page 263) for online access information for these agencies.

You can use the sites in the box to find local adult day care centers, home health agencies, residential facilities, physicians, Medicare-related insurance plans, hospitals, hospice groups, and even your local health care ombudsman. You can also use the following local resources:

- *Your doctor:* He or she may have a list of trusted agencies.
- *The Yellow Pages:* This can be a little like playing Russian roulette—you cannot be sure the center you chose will be a good one. However, the Yellow Pages can be helpful for finding phone numbers and the locations of agencies already recommended.

- *The local Area Agency on Aging:* The staff can help you sort out what you need and how to find the services.

- *Senior centers in your area:* They may have staff or volunteers available to help you find services.

- *The hospital social worker:* If you start your search in the hospital, the social worker staff can be of great help.

- *Other LBD caregivers:* This is where you may get the best and most specific answers. Your physician may be able to connect you with other LBD caregivers, or there may be an LBD support group in your area.

Your Medical Team

Because LBD is a multifaceted disease, you will likely find yourself dealing with several physicians, specialists, and other medical personnel.

> Make a calendar or date book your constant companion. When you enter your appointments, always add a phone number. This will help you if you need to call to change an appointment or for any other reason.

- *Physicians:* Your primary care physician is the doctor you will see the most. This person should be open to information about Lewy body dementia if he or she is not already LBD savvy. The primary physician will then refer you to other specialists, such as an internist or urologist and certainly a neurologist or other dementia specialist. If your loved one has Parkinson's disease (PD), you may already have a movement specialist.

- *Pharmacists:* The pharmacist is your "go-to guy" for medications. Therefore, you want one who is LBD savvy, even if you have to travel farther to get your prescriptions filled.

- *Therapists:* The primary care physician may refer your loved one to a speech therapist to help with swallowing, or to a physical therapist to learn how to relax muscles. In situations like this, you will likely be the one doing the learning so that you can help your loved one do the daily exercises. Therefore, make sure the therapist is one that you can work with.

- *Nurses and other medical staff:* Wherever you go, be it the doctor's office, a testing center, the therapist's office, the hospital emergency room, the hospital proper, or a residential facility, you will meet nurses, technicians, and aides. Often these people have little or no knowledge of LBD.

Building an LBD-Savvy Team

Chapter 2 covered how to find LBD-savvy, or at least LBD-supportive, specialists and physicians. However, your work does not stop there. You will continually have to make certain that the medical people who come into contact with your loved one are aware and supportive of the unique problems that LBD brings. To discover whether the medical people who will be working with your loved one are LBD savvy, you should do the following:

- Ask the same questions you might ask a physician concerning LBD (see Chapter 2).

- Ask what courses on LBD they have taken or if they have completed one of the credited trainings that are available for most professionals in their fields.

- Be ready to teach. Keep your wallet card (see Chapter 8) and LBDA brochures handy. It may be easier to train the medical support people who come into contact with your loved one than it is to find people who are already LBD savvy.

- Be willing to go to a drugstore, therapist, or hospital that is farther away if you find the staff there to be more LBD savvy.

Working With Your Team

Once you have a team of individuals whom you trust, let them do their jobs. If you have done a good job of choosing your professionals, even the ones you felt you had to teach at first should soon know more about LBD and all of its ramifications than you do. After all, they have a broader background of general medical knowledge on which to build. However, you will always be the specialist about your loved one and the unique way he expresses the disease, so save your energy for those jobs that only you can do, such as being your loved one's main support person and being his advocate by telling the specialists what worked and what did not.

Medical Treatment Facilities

Urgent Care

Neighborhood-based miniclinics are often available to deal with minor issues or emergencies such as cuts, headaches, or infections. If your loved one has many urinary tract infections (UTIs), urgent care may be a good resource—just do not count on the staff being LBD savvy. Bring your LBDA wallet card and be prepared to advocate for any special care or handling your loved one needs. These clinics will seldom be able to deal with most LBD-related problems, such as dehydration or extreme acting out. Therefore, except for very basic issues, like a UTI, your loved one will probably be referred to an emergency room, resulting in a very long wait at the urgent care center followed by another long wait in the emergency room.

> Unless you know your loved one is suffering from something that an urgent care facility can handle, you are better off going to a hospital emergency room.

Hospitals and Emergency Rooms

As many of us have learned the hard way, not all hospitals have LBD-savvy staff. This is especially true in their emergency rooms, the most likely place for your loved one to receive LBD-dangerous drugs. However, LBD is a disease that often expresses itself physically, in UTIs, dehydration, falls, and other problems that need emergency medical attention. Therefore, it is very likely that your loved one will make many emergency room visits and/or be hospitalized several times before his journey with this disease is over.

One advantage of going to an urgent care center as a first step is that they know more about what the hospitals in your area offer and can often refer you to the one best-suited to your problem. However, this is not necessarily true for your loved one with LBD. The special care he needs is not obvious. However, prior to any emergencies, you can research yourself which local hospitals are LBD savvy. Then your loved one will get the best care your area can provide.

To find the best hospital, talk with your dementia specialist. Ideally, you will already have found a specialist that you like. Ask this specialist which hospitals he or she works with and which is his or her favorite for patients with LBD and why. In most cases, this is the hospital you will want to go to even if it is not the one closest to you and even if the reason for hospitalization is not LBD related. Everything becomes LBD related for the person with this disease, just as Anique's ER visit to treat dehydration quickly turned LBD-related when she was given haloperidol (Haldol).

Hospitals associated with teaching and research centers are often a good place to find LBD-savvy staff. These facilities tend to offer the most up-to-date services and staff trained in the "new" diseases. Find teaching and research centers in your area by asking your specialist or your primary care physician about them.

Keeping Your Loved One at Home

During the first years of LBD, you should be able to keep your loved one at home. Some caregivers are able to do so until the very end. However, you can do a better job of caregiving and fight isolation if you use some of the home care options that are available.

Adult Day Care Centers

Adult day care centers provide social, medical, and emotional support for people with dementia and a respite for caregivers. Such a place may be able to provide the help you need if you have concluded that you cannot leave your loved one alone anymore but you are not ready to consider a residential placement.

> I still have to earn a living. Months ago, I became concerned about leaving Jake at home alone. I never knew what he might do. Once I came home from work and he had made a terrible mess in the kitchen. He'd decided to bake muffins, he told me. He quit and got involved in a TV show before he'd done more than coat the kitchen with flour. The oven was on but, thank goodness, nothing was in it. I was afraid that next time he'd try to cook something on the stovetop and burn the house down.
>
> —*Norma*

Norma had a choice of bringing in a caregiver or finding a safe place for Jake to stay while she was at work. This is a difficult time for a family. Often it is some sort of scary event, like Jake's muffins, that causes the family to realize that their loved one can no longer be left alone. Remember that LBD is different from Alzheimer's disease (AD). Jake appeared perfectly normal most of the time; however, he could fall into a bout of confusion, where he would make poor judgments and dangerous choices, at any time.

> When I suggested to Jake that maybe we should get someone to come and keep him company during the day, he told me he didn't need a babysitter. Rather than fight that battle, I decided to research adult day care centers. Jake was still alert most of the time then, so I thought this would be ideal for him. He's always been a social person and after he retired, he was alone way too much anyway.
>
> —*Norma*

These programs are a good resource for the caregiver who must work outside the home or for a caregiver who needs a few hours of daily respite. They offer structured activities, social interaction, and good nutrition for well-functioning persons with LBD. Your loved one should be continent and ambulatory, although someone who gets around well in a wheelchair would likely be accepted.

> One of the things my Harry and I agreed upon very early in his disease was that he'd go to an adult care center several times a week so that I could take some regular time away from home. He said he'd rather do that while he could than have someone come in. We both looked for a center in our area, and Harry started going about once a week at first. We found one that provides transportation, so he goes every weekday now for a few hours. He really looks forward to it.
>
> —*Nell*

Prior to selecting a care center, make a list of your loved one's specific needs. Think about things like whether you need transportation and what hours you want your loved one at the center. Request fliers from centers in your area and, after reading up on each location, tour the centers in person. Pay attention to the following, and do not be afraid to ask questions:

- Is the facility cheerful, clean, and free of odors? Is the furniture comfortable, sturdy, and the right height for easy access?

- What conditions are accepted (e.g., dementia, limited mobility, incontinence)?

- What services and activities do they offer? There should be a daily exercise program, some activities that provide mental stimulation, and some that encourage social interaction.

- What is the cost? Look for any hidden fees, such as extra charges for transportation or meals.

- Do they offer any financial assistance? Does the center know of any financial assistance from the government or elsewhere that you might be eligible for?

- What is their validation: years of service, facility and staff credentials, and so forth? Look for stability and competency.

- Pay close attention to the staff.
  - What is the ratio of staff to participants?
  - Do the staff look harried?
  - Are the staff friendly?
  - Do the staff treat people with dementia with respect?
  - Do the staff have time to sit and visit with participants or play games with them?
  - Do the staff show compassion and patience when dealing with participants?
  - Do the staff appear to be knowledgeable about the participants and their care?

- What is expected of you?
  - Must you drop off your loved one only at specific times?
  - Does the center welcome drop-ins?
  - Are you expected to volunteer? Can you volunteer if you want to?
  - Are you welcome to visit unannounced?
  - Are you expected to send a lunch or other items with your loved one?

- Do they offer transportation?
  - Does it go to your area? Is it door to door? Is it only at certain times?

- What are their hours of operation?
  - Do these hours fit your needs?
  - Do they have a policy for when you are late and cannot get to the facility until after their closing time?
  - Do they have a policy for when you need to drop off your loved one early?
- Do they have a system for helping participants transition into their program?
- Are meals and snacks included? Look at the menu. Does it meet your loved one's special needs? Did they ask you to stay for lunch? (A good sign.)

Moreover, ask the staff supervisor LBD-related questions:

- How many of your participants have LBD? The more they have, the more likely this is a good place for your loved one.
- Have your staff had LBD-specific training? Few staff members at adult day care centers do, but find out if the center is willing to offer LBD training, or at least if they are willing to encourage their staff to listen to you and read your literature.
- How does the center deal with acting-out behaviors? You want a facility with a staff that understands and uses behavior management.
- What does the staff know about fluctuating cognition? You want staff that know your loved one is not faking during a period of confusion.

Check references by talking to people who have used the center. A good center will have a list of family members who will be happy to talk to you about their own experiences with the facility. Try to talk to at least one caregiver of someone with LBD.

Once you have found an adult day care center that you like, talk to your loved one about it, and take him for a visit.

I think a part of Jake knew that it wasn't safe for him to stay alone anymore. But we didn't talk about that. Instead, we talked about how it would be so much more pleasant for him to have a nice hot meal every day for lunch and people to visit with.

—Norma

Norma focused on the things Jake liked—food and a chance to visit with people—instead of trying to fight any resistance he might have.

> I asked Jake to go with me to visit the center. We went a couple of times and I even left him there while I went shopping. That was an easy one. Jake was quite willing to wait in that nice, comfortable place and visit with those friendly people while I shopped—he's always hated going shopping with me. And then, once he found it wasn't so bad, I got him to agree to try being there during work hours "for awhile."
>
> —*Norma*

Norma took it in steps: some short visits with her along; a couple of hours without her; and, finally, a discussion about going there when Norma was at work.

> After a month, Jake adjusted. I think he liked going somewhere every day, like he was going to work too, you know. In fact, that's what he called it. The center staff was wonderful. Right away, they asked him to help and actually gave him jobs to do. And then they told him they needed help the next day and asked him if he could come back. It sucked him right in! Now, he hates missing a day. It has been a blessing for both of us. It gives Jake a sense of being useful and I don't worry about leaving him home alone.
>
> —*Norma*

Remember that it may take several visits before your loved one adjusts. However, caregivers repeatedly say that their loved ones get as much out of day care as the caregiver does, and that, like Jake, once they get used to the schedule, they enjoy going.

You can help your loved one to adjust to attending an adult day care center by doing the following:

- Going with your loved one to visit several times, staying longer each time;
- Looking for things to praise, such as good food or an especially enjoyable activity;
- Asking your loved one to stay there while you run a few errands; and
- Praising your loved one's ability to help other participants or the staff.

Home Health Care

A home health care worker comes into your home and helps you take care of your loved one. Agencies can provide full-time or part-time staff, depending on what you want. The home care staff may include not only aides but also nurses, physical therapists, speech therapists, and social workers. They may also have a social worker who can help you find other resources, such as financial guidance or legal help. There are also unaffiliated individuals who do this work, but they may not be as easy to find as an agency—and they may be more difficult to check into.

> When Anique came home from the hospital, we had to have home health aides around the clock. That only lasted for a short time, until Anique felt a bit better and I'd mastered how to do the job. Then I decreased their time to just 4 hours three times a week.
>
> *—Jim*

Often, a caregiver like Jim will have no idea of how to be a spouse's nurse. The health aides provided the care Anique needed while he learned. Once he felt competent to do the job, he cut back, but he did not stop having them come altogether. The few hours a week that the workers came in allowed Anique to have a woman's help at bath time and gave Jim a chance to go shopping and just get out of the house for a while. Respite is a very important aspect of caregiving but is often overlooked.

Home health care has several advantages:

- Your loved one can stay in his own home.
- The care is one on one—he does not have to wait his turn.
- It is usually less expensive than residential care (unless he requires 'round-the-clock care).

Hospice

Hospice is a free service for anyone on Medicare who meets the hospice criteria. It provides palliative (pain-easing) care that includes nursing, assistance with personal care, some medications, hospital beds, canes, and other supplies that your loved one might need. Many people think hospice is just for the very last days of one's life. However, when your loved one has dementia, the rules are different; he must be fairly helpless but does not have to be dying to go on hospice. Hospice services will usually make it possible for you to keep your loved one at home much longer than you otherwise could. Hospice services, including the requirements for someone with dementia to be able to receive this free care, are covered more completely in Chapter 14.

Making the Decision

The decision to start home health care may be initiated by some crisis that changes the persons' ability to care for themselves, such as surgery or a bad fall. People with dementia who have home care can be much less physically and/or cognitively functional than those who go to adult care centers.

> We had several health aides come in before we found one that we both liked. Once we found Rosalie, we asked for her regularly.
>
> —*Howard*

It may be that Howard was resisting the need for help by saying that Emma did not like the health aides. It is not easy to accept that it is not possible to do everything alone. The health aide becomes a part of the family while she is there. She needs to be someone who is compatible not only with your loved one but also with you.

> My dad lives about a mile from us. I wish I could just move in with him, but I have my own family to consider. We thought about having him move in with us, but we don't have room and he is adamant about living in his own home anyway. We've worked it out so that one of us is with him most of the time. I am there most days but our son, Leon, sleeps there and our daughter, Bernice, spends Sundays with her grandpa. We know it's important not to burn out so we have a health aide for about 4 hours every evening and all day Saturday. On her days off, either my husband goes over and has a "guy night" with Dad or Dad comes here. This works for now, but we know the time will come when we'll have to have more help.
>
> —*Kyla, daughter of Ed*

Many families share responsibilities as Kyla and her family do. However, this is usually a short-term solution. As Kyla said, they will probably eventually need to consider residential care.

When my sister Lucille became ill with cancer, I had just retired and was able to move in with her and be her full-time caregiver. I had worked in the health field throughout my career, so I knew how important respite was to someone who is both a caregiver and a loved one. Therefore, we agreed right at the start that Lucille would hire a respite caregiver every 2 weeks so that I could have a few days off. Lucille and I did not go through an agency but found an individual, recommended to us by a friend whom I trusted. You can find individual caregivers by doing the following:

- Asking other people, especially other families with caregiver needs. This is often best because it provides a built-in reference.

- Asking doctors or other professionals such as the nurses and social workers.

- Looking in the paper for ads.

No matter how you find your caregiver, be sure to ask for references and then check them out.

My sister Lucille's caregiver, Rosa, was competent, pleasant, and had religious beliefs similar to Lucille's. This last was important because my sister had been a missionary. Like most invalids, my once-gregarious sister had become more and more isolated as her illness increased. Rosa was a new face, and she and my sister started out with something in common that was important to both of them.

Such cultural issues can be very important. A person cared for at home may be more isolated than if they are in a residential facility where people are coming and going all day. Most of the people they will meet at home will be in some way related to their illness: the respite caregivers, visiting nurses, social workers, and even the pastor who is making sick calls. This is especially true if the primary caregiver cannot drive or cannot safely get her loved one in or out of a vehicle. If your loved one has anything he feels strongly about, like Lucille and her religion, choosing a home care helper with similar beliefs or hobbies will give them an immediate area of compatibility. Perhaps politics or sports are your loved one's passion. The more areas of compatibility you can find culturally, the easier it will be for your loved one to accept and enjoy this new person.

When choosing a helper, identify the tasks you want the helper to do. If any of these tasks involve specialized nursing care, you will need a licensed practical nurse (LPN) or a registered nurse (RN). Otherwise, you can hire a skilled helper, which will be much less expensive.

It is important for your loved one to feel that he had some say in the final decision. However, participating in the interviews would be much too stressful. Do them yourself and narrow the field down to a couple of choices. Then hire the one you like the most to come to work for a few hours, and ask your loved one what he thinks about the one you hired. If he is undecided or does not like this one, then ask your second-choice worker to come. This way, your loved one can choose which one he likes best.

During your interviews, you may want to ask the following questions:

- Do you offer the services we need, such as:
  - Personal care, which might include help with transfers from bed to chair, bathing, dressing, and toileting? Can you do the lifting required?
  - (For nurses) IV insertion, catheterization, wound care, and so forth?
  - Housekeeping, such as cooking, cleaning, and laundry? It is a good idea to agree ahead of time on what nonpatient care jobs the individual will be expected to do.
  - Transportation, to places such as shopping and doctor visits? Who provides the vehicle?
- Can you meet our special needs, such as language, religious, or cultural preferences? (Know ahead of time what these special needs are and ask specific questions about them.)
- What hours are you available? Can you work the hours when we need help? Are you available to stay if I want to be gone overnight?
- How much do you know about Lewy body dementia? Are you willing to learn about the special issues of dealing with a person with this disease? (Not knowing about LBD should not be a deal breaker as long as the person is willing to learn.)

- Do you use behavior management techniques? (If the person does not, there will likely be more behavior problems. Unlike sharing information about LBD, trying to teach a helper about behavior management is more than the average family caregiver will want to take on.)
- Can you provide references? (Make sure at least one of the references is from a family who has a loved one with dementia, if not LBD.)

If you want to use an agency, these are some of the ways you can find one in your area[7]:

- Visit the Medicare site (see Online References, Page 263).
- Ask your doctor, hospital discharge planner, or friends and family.
- Use a senior referral service.
- Look in the Yellow Pages under "home care" or "home health care."

Ask questions similar to those you would ask an individual caregiver. In addition, ask questions such as the following:

- Is the same person assigned to us each time? Can we ask for a change if my loved one does not do well with the first one you send? (This might be a deal breaker if they do not. It is difficult enough for your loved one to get used to one new person, let alone several.)
- Does the agency offer extra services for speech or physical therapy? Do the therapists come to our home or do we go to them?
- Do you have staff available to provide the type and hours of care that we need?
- Do you have staff available at night and weekends for emergencies?
- Are you Medicare certified? What will Medicare and/or my insurance cover, and what expenses must we pay?
- Are background checks performed on all staff members?
- Do you have references who testify that your staff provide good care?

In addition, you need to ask some LBD-specific questions such as:

- How much training about Lewy body dementia do you provide your staff? (If none, request that any staff member assigned to your loved one becomes trained via readings that you provide.)
- How do you handle behavior problems and acting out? Are your staff trained in behavior management techniques?
- What does the staff know about fluctuating cognition? (You want to know that the workers will use the *good times* and will not think your loved one is faking the *bad times*.)
- What do your staff know about LBD drug sensitivities and the symptoms to look for? (The sooner adverse symptoms are noticed, the better.)

As with an individual caregiver, you should choose only one agency at a time for your loved one to approve.

Quick Tip

Have a new helper come when your loved one is most aware (during a *good time*). He will be most able to deal with change then. Even though your loved one may not seem to recognize the new worker the next time she comes, a part of him will, making him more accepting.

It may take awhile for your loved one to accept a worker in your home to the extent that he feels safe without you there. Plan to stay home the first few times anyone comes. This will also give you a chance to evaluate the new worker's skill.

Sometimes you must make a decision between home health care and residential care.

I'm just not able to care for Emma anymore. My doctor told me I couldn't do the lifting because of my heart. He said that if I couldn't find someone to come help me, I'd have to put Emma into residential care.

—Howard

A huge advantage of home care is that Howard and Emma can stay in their own home, something that both of them prefer. Home care often works quite well if it is needed for only a few hours a week. However, it may not be practical for this couple, who likely need 24-hour coverage. The multiple shifts and the larger variety of people in their home would be confusing for Emma and could become overwhelming for Howard. For instance, if someone does not show up or calls in sick, then Howard would be alone for that shift unless someone else were found to cover. He may be better off considering residential care of some sort.

Caregivers of a person with dementia with Lewy bodies (DLB), that is, dementia without movement problems, may believe that because there are fewer mobility issues they will be able to keep their loved one at home indefinitely. This is not necessarily so. Other issues can make home care impractical or even unsafe.

> Early in her illness, Anique begged me to promise I'd never put her in a nursing home. At that time, I had no hesitation making such a promise. She had mental problems, but physically she was fine, and I didn't see why this wouldn't continue. Then, in the last months of her illness, Anique became so delusional and combative that I couldn't keep her at home, even with around-the-clock help. This decision was very difficult for me and it was even worse because Anique couldn't understand why I wasn't keeping my promise to her. But I had no choice. It just wasn't safe.
>
> —*Jim*

Jim had unknowingly made a common caregiver's mistake: He made a promise he could not keep, and then Anique felt betrayed. She never forgave him. It is understandable that our loved ones will try to get us to promise to keep them at home. For them, it is bad enough to feel that they are losing control of their lives. To lose one's home as well must seem intolerable. However, you are doing your loved one— and yourself—no favors if you make this often-impossible-to-keep promise.

People are different. Our friend Bill dealt better with the future when he knew what to expect. If your loved one is like this, we hope you are reading this early in his disease. After the diagnosis, while he is still able to reason, sit down together and discuss the future as soon as possible. Talk about the possibility that the time may come when you will not be able to care for him safely. Discuss alternative plans for care. Have him participate in the choice of a facility, or, if that is not possible, discuss why a care facility is most important for his health and safety. For instance, is an outside space high on his list of priorities or simply nice? Caregivers report that later, when difficult choices are necessary, their loved ones accept better those decisions they once discussed—even when they no longer remember doing so.

Other people are like Anique: They see discussing the future and the challenges it may hold as an acceptance of the unacceptable. They may ask you to promise to keep them at home "no matter what." Do not set them, and yourself, up for future pain. A decision for residential care will be difficult enough, even if it is quite necessary. However, your loved ones will be more accepting of the decision if they are not holding on to a promise that was impossible to keep, and you will feel less guilty. That sense of guilt harms not only you but also your loved ones. They can sense it and will feel even more justified in their anger at you for "betraying" them.

If Anique had had Alzheimer's disease, she would never have remembered that promise. However, with LBD, some memories last—and for Anique that promise was one she never forgot. Of course, what did not last was her ability to make rational judgments.

> Never make a promise you cannot keep. "I'll keep you at home as long as I safely can" is the most you should promise. No matter what your health or your loved one's condition is now things can change quickly into a situation where it may no longer be safe to care for your loved one at home.

Finances may be another deciding issue. Although a few hours a week of home care is usually much less expensive than residential care, 24-hour home care may be more expensive. This may come up when several family members are sharing expenses.

> Our sons have been paying for a health aide come in to stay with Harry a few hours a week so I can go shopping and such. I think that's all we need for now. But the kids say we need more, and they want him to go into a dementia care center. They say it will be cheaper than paying for the home health aide—that we could sell our house and use the proceeds to pay for the residential care. Well, they may be right, and eventually we might do that. But we aren't ready for such a big change yet.
> —*Nell*

Nell probably needs an expert, perhaps a social worker from the home health agency that provides their helper, to come evaluate their situation. If Nell is right, and it is safe for her to provide the care when there is no one else there, she might consider doing a reverse mortgage, so that she gets a payment each month to help with expenses. This would allow them to live in their home but still have extra funds (see Chapter 13).

Residential Facilities

Residential settings vary from an independent living situation, in which the residents are very self-sufficient, to a nursing home, where the residents may be able do very little for themselves. Many facilities are multilevel, meaning that they offer housing with several levels of assistance, depending on the needs of the resident. This is very attractive to a couple who, although they are still self-sufficient, know that eventually they are going to need more help. Living in a multilevel facility allows them to move to a level with more assistance without leaving their friends or activities.

Independent Living

To qualify for this level, a person or couple needs to be very self-sufficient. A big attraction for this kind of living is the decreased isolation. Many organized activities, such as bingo, painting, or card playing, make it easy to socialize. There are usually dining facilities and health support right in the building. If you are considering an apartment in a multilevel facility as a first step toward more care later on, be sure to check out what the other levels of care offer and how LBD supportive they are.

Assisted Care

To live in an assisted care apartment, residents must be able to live safely without continual care. It is not much different than having a home health care worker come in for a few hours a day except that the help can be spread out over the whole day instead of all at one time. The staff are available to help with bedtimes and getting up, and possibly with toileting. Residents are expected to go to the dining room for certain meals, with assistance if needed, but can prepare and eat other meals in their rooms if they prefer. The same activities and outings are offered to people in assisted care as to those in independent care.

Caregiver spouses often choose to go into assisted living situations with their loved ones when they become unable to do the heavier caregiving jobs anymore. That way, the couple can remain together, but there is a staff to help with toileting and other lifting needs. The largest assisted care apartments may have two bedrooms but only one bedroom is more common and many are studio apartments. Therefore, housekeeping chores become much less demanding. To balance the small living space and as a way to encourage residents not to isolate, these facilities offer large public areas for socializing and eating. They also offer many organized activities, from church, to card playing, to hobbies such as painting, and well-filled libraries for reading.

Dementia Care

The dementia care part of a residential facility is usually designed more with safety in mind than standard of living.[8] Often, it is a locked wing with an open courtyard in the center, so that residents can go outside without the danger of wandering off. Although wandering is less a problem with LBD than with AD, it can happen and needs to be safeguarded against. Because people with dementia get disoriented easily, there will likely be a very simple floor plan. All meals are prepared by the facility staff because cooking involves too many hazards. Staff in this level of care should be well trained in the use of behavior management.

Nursing Home Care

When persons become so physically debilitated that they can no longer do very much for themselves, then a nursing home may become an option. The need for a nursing home often comes on suddenly, after a crisis that seriously decreases your loved one's ability to function. For a person with dementia, this is often an end-of-life decision and may not be needed if there is a good hospice program available in your community. However, if this level of care should be needed, the qualifications of the staff become much more important.

> Choose a facility that is easy for you to visit. Even in excellent facilities, the residents with the most frequent visitors are the ones who receive the best care.

Searching for a Residential Facility

You can start your search well in advance by contacting your community's long-term care ombudsman[9] and by asking about the laws, regulations, and licensing requirements for residential facilities in your state. Even if you are at present interested only in assisted living care, ask about dementia care and nursing home care requirements as well. You may not ever need these, but if you do you will want to have the information available. These requirements will tell you the basic services that each type of facility must provide and qualifications they must meet. Qualifications will vary with the level of care a facility requires. Each facility should have its licenses prominently posted.

You will want to research residential facilities in a way similar to that discussed in the section about adult day care centers. It will help if you make up a list of questions to ask before you go so you will not forget anything. Start with the list of questions about adult care centers. Then add some of the following questions as well.

Questions for an Assisted Living Facility

- Are the staff's attitude toward medication the same as mine? As the level of care increases, so do the staff's control of the resident's medications. Many drugs are given on an "as needed" basis. Make sure that their attitude toward medicating for behavior control matches your own and that they do not use medications known to be unsafe with LBD (see Chapter 8).

- Does the facility have a memory care program for slowing down the progress of dementia? It should include exercise, socialization, and mental stimulation.

- Does the facility have a nutritional department that serves brain-healthy food in an attractive way?

- Is there an emphasis on allowing residents to be as independent as possible? Do the staff take into consideration that your loved one's ability to function varies from day to day because of fluctuating cognition?

- Ask to see the resident's bill of rights. Do the staff include a copy of this with the intake papers when a person becomes a resident of their facility?

- What kind of safety devices and precautions do you see? Are there handrails in bathing areas and hallways? Are halls and doors wide? Are the floors neither slippery nor heavily carpeted? Are exits marked clearly?

Questions for a Dementia Care Center

(Note that necessary safety issues can lead to somewhat different answers to the general questions.)

- How does the facility act to prevent abuse? There should be a process of some sort, like regular supervision of the staff at work and a formal report procedure for families to use as needed.
- How do staff balance the need to keep residents safe and contained with quality-of-life issues such as comfort and self-respect? For instance, is there an enclosed outdoor area?
- How is the family included in treatment? There should be weekly or at least monthly meetings between family members and staff to plan treatment.
- Are there things that you can and cannot do? For instance, insurance issues often prevent anyone other than staff from doing any lifting. Or, if your loved one is on a special diet, you may not be allowed to bring in extra food. If you disagree with any of these regulations, the best time to question them is before your loved one moves in.

Questions for a Nursing Home[10]

- What kind of training do their staff receive? Make sure that at least some of the training addresses working with people who have Lewy body dementia, or that the staff are open for you to teach them how to work with your loved one.
- How many of the staff are trained nurses (licensed vocational nurses [LVNs], LPNs, or RNs) and how many are nursing care assistants?
- Is there a social worker on staff? A physician? How accessible are they to residents and family?

- How many licensed RNs are on staff at all times? Is there a time when the RN is not present but is on call only?
- Do they have lifting devices so the staff do not have to lift residents manually?
- Is the floor plan such that ambulatory residents have only a short distance to go for dining and activities?

Day-to-Day Residential Living

Once you have chosen a facility, talk to the staff about your expectations and theirs.

> Before we put Mom into a dementia care center, I talked to the director of nurses. We agreed on a schedule that worked for Mom and fit with the facility's schedule. Mom couldn't have everything the same as we'd had it at home, but I knew going in that she'd have the important things, like the medications that she needs at times when they worked best for her. I made sure I could still help with Mom's care. The director explained that there were certain things that I couldn't do because of insurance—like lifting her on and off the toilet— but that the aides would welcome my help in other ways. Knowing ahead of time what I could and couldn't do saved me a lot of frustration later on. And having the aides know at the beginning that I expected to be a part of the treatment team helped too.
>
> —*Marion, daughter of Clara*

By recruiting the director's help before placement and making sure the director knew her mother's special needs, Marion felt herself to be a part of the care team from the start. With the guidance from the director, the care providers also knew what to expect from Marion and worked with her from the beginning.

Abuse Issues

Abuse becomes more common as residents become less able to communicate. Your loved one may not remember to complain to you or he may be paranoid and complain about everything, making it difficult to know whether abuse is really happening. A staff who are well trained in behavior management can be a deterrent of abuse but not a guarantee that it is not happening. Abuse is also an issue in nursing homes, where debilitated residents are at the mercy of staff both physically and emotionally. Thus, frequent visits become very important. With these issues in mind, a facility near your home may be a better choice than a nicer one that is farther away.

Fitting In

If you want your loved one to be content in this new situation, you will have to adjust to this new situation yourself as well. Unless you do, your loved one will continue to reflect your feelings and will not be able to adjust either. No one says this is easy, but it is imperative that you find a way to accept the changes.

Caregivers often feel guilty when they must place their loved one into a residential setting. They may also feel that they have become useless and unneeded now that someone else is physically caring for their loved one.

> I shudder to think how bossy I was when Peter was first put into the dementia care wing. I had to tell the aide everything. I didn't like the way they made the bed; I hated how the meals were served. . . . But when I began to see the care providers as part of our team instead of opponents, Peter started getting much better care. I learned to let them do their job and focus only on the ways I could help Peter. For instance, only I knew that Peter would take his meds better with pudding instead of applesauce. He doesn't like apples but he loves chocolate!
>
> —*Jenny*

As caregiver in a residential setting your job is that of advocate, support person, and expert on your loved one's unique expression of this disease. No one else can do these jobs as well as you can. Let go of the guilt, and see that by placing your loved one in a residential home you are still doing your job to the best of your ability. You have not deserted him, and you still have great value, not only to him but also to those who now perform his physical care.

Isolation

A newly placed person, especially someone with dementia, may have a very difficult time relating to all the new people and activities. Unless family is there to encourage them, it is much easier to remain isolated. Therefore, much of your time at first will likely be spent taking your loved one out of his room so he can be where other people are, taking him to activities so he can participate, eating with him, and generally helping him to become acclimated to the facility. Staff will also be there to help with these activities, but it is not the same, especially at first. With you at his side, your loved one has some continuity and will be more able to deal with all of the new and confusing routines, people, and activities.

There are a few ways you can make residential living a better experience for both you and your loved one:

- Spend as much time as possible in the facility, and vary the times you visit. Consider volunteering so that you become an actual part of the staff. However, do not spend all of your time there. Take some time to care for yourself.

- Bring a few of your loved one's personal items to display in his room. It will make the place seem more like home.

- Continue to keep a diary. Although it is true that the residential facility will also be keeping a record of some sort about your loved one, do not count on it being as thorough or as focused on LBD issues, such as fluctuations, as yours will be.

- Help the staff get to know your loved one better by sharing details about his personal history, likes and dislikes, and preferred routines. Show how certain behavior management techniques work better with your loved one than others.

- Speak up when you have concerns. To assist with later investigations, use your diary to document problems you observe (date, time, staff involved, and any other witnesses). This will give your complaints much more validity and help the facility make needed changes. Concerns should be voiced first to the supervisor, not to the hands-on staff. If there is not an improvement, then go to the supervisor again and demand a change, such as different staff or a different room. If a similar problem occurs the third time, consider going to your ombudsman.

- Participate in any family council meetings or care plan conferences that are offered, and then follow up to see that the plan is being followed. Request a meeting with the supervisor if it is not.

- Educate the staff about Lewy body dementia. Offer to share books and articles, and recommend Internet Web pages, such as the LBDA Web site.

- Accompany your loved one to activities and meals. He will enjoy it more with you along, and the more you know about his schedule, the better. It is especially important for you to accompany your loved one to therapist's appointments and the like. Because learning is a lost art for your loved one, he will need help and guidance to do the daily exercises. Naturally, that will be part of the staff's duties, but if you learn the exercises you can also help.

- Compliment the staff every chance you get, and always report excellent care to supervisors. This makes the staff's job more pleasant—and they will do a better job for your loved one. Sometimes, facilities have contests in which the staff person with the most positive comments wins a prize. Support such practices; they improve your loved one's care.

Finally, as much as possible, make yourself at home in the facility. Learn what you can and cannot do. Learn about the amenities. Is there a small kitchen area where you can get coffee or heat something in the microwave? A room with a big table where you and your loved one can do some scrapbooking? Is there a best time for you and your loved one to go for a walk? Get to know the staff members who care for your loved one. You are "coworkers," caring for the same person. These people will become your loved one's family in many ways. Support them and help them to give the best care they can.

13

Managing Legal and Financial Issues

When a person is diagnosed with Lewy body dementia (LBD), legal issues become important. If the person is a spouse who has been the one in charge of family finances and legal issues, this will have to change. Ideally, the couple will discuss these issues while the person with LBD can still be a part of the planning process. That's what Nell and her husband Harry did.

> We decided that we would make sure everything was in joint ownership. That way, I'd be able to sign checks and legal documents when I needed to.
>
> *—Nell*

Joint ownership is a good start. Make certain that the caregiver's name is the primary one on the account so that she has access to all important information. Depending on bank policies, it may be necessary to open a new account. If you bank online, write down the account ID and passwords in a safe place.

> We weren't sure what else to do, and we decided to find a lawyer to help us instead.
>
> *—Nell*

A lawyer is an excellent idea; financial and legal decisions for most LBD families can be quite confusing. An elder law attorney is the best choice; he or she will be more aware of the legal needs of the LBD family. If cost is an issue, community senior centers often offer free legal consultations. Contact your local Agency on Aging office or the Eldercare Locator for more information.

Our budget is so tight; I didn't see how we could afford a lawyer. I was just going to try to do it all myself, somehow. They have forms on the Internet, you know. But when I mentioned that to my support group, they all insisted that I needed a lawyer. One woman who'd been through it all told me, "Even if you have to go without something or let the rent get behind, you HAVE to have a lawyer. Too many things can happen that you might not even consider." So I went to the senior center and talked to a fellow there, a retired lawyer that donated his time once a week. He recommended an elder care lawyer who was willing to take payments.

—Howard

Caregivers emphatically recommend an attorney to guide you in making the right decisions and getting the proper documents in order. One or two visits are usually enough.

Advance Directives

In addition to joint bank accounts, there are several other financial and legal documents to consider while your loved one is still able to make decisions. An attorney can explain in more detail, but here is a very brief rundown[1]:

- *Power of attorney (POA):* There are several different kinds, all allowing you to act on your loved one's behalf.
  - *Basic POA:* This will not benefit the LBD family because it is valid only when your loved one still has the mental capacity to make decisions.
  - *Springing POA:* Although an attractive option for individuals who are not ready give up control of their affairs, the springing POA is not a very good choice for the LBD family. For this POA to become effective, your loved one must be proven unable to make his own decisions. A diagnosis of dementia alone is not adequate; *incompetency* must also be reported. Examining physicians who do not know about LBD's fluctuating cognition may not be able to see enough evidence to make such a drastic judgment, especially if your loved one puts on his best *showtime* behavior during an examination.

- *Durable POA:* This option becomes active immediately and lasts until death, although it can be revoked by your loved ones as long as they are still capable of making decisions. A durable power of attorney is usually the best type for an LBD family. With this, a caregiver can gradually take over financial and legal tasks.

- *General POA and health care POA:* These can each be basic, springing or durable, but they cover only certain areas of your loved one's affairs. A general POA covers all financial and legal issues, and a health POA covers medical issues. Your lawyer will probably recommend separate general and health care powers of attorney.

- *Living will:* The living will provides information for end-of-life decisions. This document helps immensely because it makes your loved one's wishes plain to everyone. Hospitals now request that all patients have a health care directive, which includes a living will, on file.

- *Will:* This document directs how one's worldly goods are to be distributed after death. Both you and your loved one should make or review your wills soon after he is diagnosed with LBD. Discuss whom he would want as his caregiver if something were to happen to you, and include his wishes about this in your will. This way, if he is no longer able to communicate his preferences, they will still be observed. "Who will care for my loved one if I cannot?" is an issue that caregivers agonize over constantly. Making plans ahead will stop much of this worry.

- *Living trust:* This is somewhat like a combination durable power of attorney and will for financial and legal matters only. It names a "trustee"—the caregiver or someone else—to carefully invest and manage the property (assets) of the trust. Your loved one must be able make his own financial decisions at the time the document is created, but it remains in effect after dementia sets in and even after death. This makes it an attractive choice for someone with early stage dementia.

- *Inventory of all assets and expenses:* If you do this early in your loved one's disease it will be easier for you to take over the job of handling his obligations later on. It will also ensure that the lawyer has the information required to prepare needed documents. Include the following:

- ○ *Bank, brokerage, and savings accounts:* If the accounts are joint, show this. Include the latest statements.
- ○ *Real estate:* Include a copy of the deeds if possible. Show any other owners. What is owed? What is the equity?
- ○ *Any other assets:* This includes valuables such as paintings or jewelry.
- ○ *A list of income sources:* Include the amount and frequency of payments.
- ○ *A list of insurance policies:* List auto, life, and health insurance, and include contracts.
- ○ *A list of active credit cards and their balance:* Who is the primary holder and who are the signers? As with bank accounts, these should be changed so that the caregiver is the primary cardholder.
- ○ *A list of regular bills:* This should cover all bills that need to be paid regularly.
- ○ *A list of irregular bills:* Bills that may come due at irregular times, such as insurances or tax payments, go on this list.
- ○ *Any other financial or legal obligations.*
- ○ *A list of important family members:* Include everyone whom your loved one will want in any documents, such as a will and their relationship to your loved one.
- ○ *Statement of health:* A statement from your loved one's physician stating that he is still capable of making decisions.

- *List of preferences:* This is similar to a living will but pertains to things other than end-of-life decisions. Include anything that is important to your loved one and his care. If you have chosen a residential facility, name it. If he wants to stay home, state that—with the caveat "as long as it is safe." This list can also include those things that might go into a will but might not be known in time to be of use, such as what kind of a memorial service he would prefer. Some people like to include a list of personal items to be given to various people. This list of preferences is not legally binding; it simply gives the caregiver some more guidance when making decisions for her loved one. And, like a living will, such directives now can cause fewer hard feelings among relatives later.

Guardianship

If you believe your loved one is no longer capable of making legal decisions, it may be time to get a court-ordered guardianship. As guardian, you can make decisions for your loved one in all areas of his life. Earlier in this book, Barney talked about signing a directive to the hospital itemizing those drugs he knew were dangerous for Hilda. He could have done this with a durable power of attorney too, but as guardian it was an even stronger statement.

To become a guardian, you must have proof that your loved one is legally incompetent. As with a springing power of attorney, this requires the testimony from at least two physicians who have examined your loved one and found him incapable of making his own decisions. *Showtime* issues may make this difficult, unless the examining physicians are LBD savvy (see Chapter 4). Therefore, if you already have a durable power of attorney you may not want to bother with this more involved step. Your attorney can help you to decide.

Now is also the time for you and the lawyer to discuss arranging for a brain autopsy. Without the brain donations from earlier LBD families the medical field would know much less about Lewy body dementia than it does. In turn, your contribution can make an enormous difference for future LBD families. Arrangements must be made well before death. A special advantage of donating your loved one's brain is that you will receive a copy of the autopsy report. Thus, if you had any question about what kind of dementia your loved one had, you will now know for sure.

I was so glad I made the effort to arrange for Dad's brain to be donated. His symptoms were so true to the definitions for Lewy body dementia that I had no doubt that that's what he had. However, what I didn't know was that he also had Alzheimer's and even some vascular dementia. I had heard that dementias seldom came in only one kind, but I'd never thought much about it. I don't think knowing it earlier would have changed anything, but it was interesting and maybe it will help someone else.

—Eleanor

You can read more about brain autopsies and the places you can contact to arrange donations on the Lewy Body Dementia Association (LBDA) Web site.[2]

When you meet with the attorney, bring financial information and an outline of what you and your loved one have decided. Also bring a list of questions such as the following:

- How do we turn individual bank accounts and other assets (such as credit cards) into jointly owned assets? What else should we do?

- Is a power of attorney, a living trust, or a guardianship best for our situation? If a POA is most suitable, is the durable POA the best for us?

- If we choose a living trust, do we need a will too? What should be in either or both of these documents?

- What should I do to make sure that my loved one is cared for if something happens to me?

- What is involved in arranging for a brain autopsy?

Making the Change

Preplanning can make this change much less painful. Getting the necessary documents signed while your loved one is still able to make sound judgments will set a smooth path for the change of responsibilities that will eventually be needed. Sometimes, this can be quite straightforward, especially with nonspouse caregivers.

When I went to live with my sister, Lucille, she was still able to get around well. We went to the bank and she added me on to her bank account as a signee. From that time on, I could write checks for her. Because she had Parkinson's disease (PD), not Parkinson's disease with dementia (PDD), that was all we needed to do financially. If she had been showing obvious signs of dementia, this would have been the time for her to also sign a durable power of attorney and make any other legal arrangements that might have been needed so that I could act for her.

In some cases, it is easy to see when such changes are necessary, as when Clara moved in with her daughter Marion, or as in the preceding situation, when I moved in with Lucille. Sometimes, however, the changes are more subtle.

Dad remained in his own home, but we stayed with him a good share of the time. When we realized he was becoming confused more often, I asked him if he'd let me be a cosigner on his checkbook. He agreed to that, and, in fact, asked me to take over doing the bills right away. That's when I suggested that it might be easier for him if he gave me a power of attorney as well. I'm sure glad we did that because if we hadn't I have had to go to court and ask for guardianship by now. As it is, I don't think I'll ever have to do that.

—*Kyla, daughter of Ed*

Ed did not resist sharing his fiscal care with Kyla, and so this was an easy transfer. The early shift of responsibilities also prevented Kyla from having to go through the process of becoming Ed's guardian later. Because Ed handed over his financial and legal affairs immediately, they did not have to worry about when she should take them over. However, it is not always that easy.

I live in a different city from Mom and can only visit now and then. The last time we visited, I talked her into going to the doctor, and he diagnosed LBD. I invited her to move to my home, where she'd have her own bedroom and bathroom, but she got angry and insisted that I just wanted her money. That's a laugh . . . all she has is the retirement Dad left and a small Social Security check. I already pay some of her utilities. She is still able to get around well, but she isn't taking care of herself, and I'm concerned about leaving her alone. Mom wouldn't sign a power of attorney, but she did agree to let me hire a "companion." Then less than a month later, she fired her. I don't know what to do.

—*Edward*

Although Edward's story is, sadly, not uncommon, there are no easy answers. He can try to get guardianship, although this may be difficult because his mother is still more aware than confused, or he can wait and let his mother get worse and hope she does not harm herself in the meantime. He can also simply continue to try to convince her that he wants her good health and not her finances but, as one caregiver said, "trying to reason with someone whose 'reasoner' is broken is usually hopeless."

With couples, your loved one's decision making will eventually become so stressful that there will be no question—he will usually give up the responsibility voluntarily. However, by that time you may have found you waited a bit too long.

> Hilda has always been the one to pay our bills, but then I discovered that the house payment was 2 months overdue. She didn't argue when I offered to take a turn at paying them. That's when I also discovered that our bank account was overdrawn because Hilda had spent the money on toys that she mailed to the grandkids. I managed to "lose" the checkbook and credit cards and put a limited amount of cash in her purse instead. Now, I try not to do our online banking and such when she's around. I've found that as long as she isn't reminded of her loss, she's fine.
>
> *—Barney*

Often the change of responsibilities does not happen until a major problem occurs, such as important bills going unpaid. A person with LBD will often be resistant to giving up these responsibilities, just as he may not want to give up his driver's license. Because a person with LBD has a limited attention span, Barney's rationale of "out of sight, out of mind" will likely work. Notice that Barney was also careful to frame the change of responsibility in a way Hilda could accept.

Once Barney took over the finances, Hilda did not want to be involved anymore. Some people with LBD react to these changes like Hilda did, by giving up all interest in control. Others give up the physical control but want to monitor the process.

> I'm at my wits' end. We've always had joint bank accounts, and David has never been critical of my spending. But now that I'm the only one writing checks, he wants me to tell him everything I've bought, and then he tells me we didn't need it or that I bought the wrong kind or makes some other derogatory remark about my spending.
>
> *—Marie*

Patience is a wonderful virtue in a situation like this because there is no real solution to Marie's dilemma. David is exerting control in the only way he feels he has left: by complaining about how his wife does a job that was once his. Caregivers say that they must continually tell themselves, "It's the disease talking, not my loved one."

At least Marie started out with a joint bank account. Jenny did not:

> After Peter fell, I tried to get him to sign for me to do the bank-ing and all, but he refused. He was in the dementia care center and obviously unable to handle our finances anymore, so I talked to the facility social worker and she told me how to become Peter's legal guardian. Now I have full control of all of our finances and real estate, and I can make decisions about his care.
>
> —*Jenny*

In Jenny's situation, in which Peter's condition degenerated very quickly after his fall, guardianship is the only answer. Even if Peter had been willing to put Jenny on their bank account, it might not have been legal because his cognition had become more confused than alert. Sometimes it is not necessary to do anything quite that drastic. Norma did it this way:

> I suggested to Jake that we both do legal, financial, and medical powers of attorney so that if anything happened to either of us, the other would be able to make decisions more easily. He went along with it, and then I took all of the paperwork and "put it away for safekeeping." I know that if it is out of sight, he'll prob-ably forget all about what I signed. If he does ask, I'll put him off by saying I'll have to get it from the bank.
>
> —*Norma*

Many caregivers have used Norma's face-saving idea of "let's both do this" successfully, then relied on the "out of sight, out of mind" aspect of LBD to protect themselves from their loved one's misuse of the documents. Nell took a different approach.

> When my Harry first began to have symptoms, we went to see the free lawyer that our local senior center provides, and he sug-gested that we make sure all of our bank accounts, credit cards, and legal papers were in both of our names with me as the pri-mary. He also suggested that Harry sign financial, legal, and med-ical powers of attorney for me, with stipulations for when they would become valid, like "when I can no longer make good deci-sions, as decided by at least two physicians." We did all of that and I'm so glad. I don't think my Harry would be so willing to give

up control now—he's had to give up so much that he's become very protective of his remaining signs of "manhood."

—*Nell*

Nell and Harry did what caregivers seriously recommend that everyone do. Do not put this off. Your loved one will seldom become more willing to make these decisions as the disease progresses and will eventually become unable to make them. If your loved ones are agreeable to making plans for the future at the beginning of their dementia journey, be sure to do so. It gives them a chance to be involved in the decision-making process, and you will have a much better idea of what their wishes are. In addition, it is likely that when the dementia gets worse, your loved one may be less willing to let go of tasks related to being an adult.

Note that Harry signed a springing power of attorney. Nell may have some difficulty getting this put into effect. If your lawyer suggests this option, explain about *showtime* and ask whether a durable power of attorney might not be better.

If your loved one is more like Anique, who remained in denial for most of her dementia journey, you may have to enter the court system and petition to become his legal guardian, as Jenny did for Peter. As the dementia increases, you may wish to do this anyway, because a person with dementia has the right to revoke a power of attorney at any time unless he has been declared incompetent. He also has the same right to do his own business even when you do not agree with his judgments.

Making Ends Meet

Dementia is an expensive disease. The medications are costly and, as the condition degenerates, the need for physical help with caregiving can escalate from a few hours a week to full-time residential care. The expense increases with LBD's physical ailments and their complications, which can require additional medications, doctors, and hospitalizations.

Financial problems may also come from decreased income. LBD is not only a disease of the elderly. When LBD strikes a person of wage-earning age, as was the case with 52-year-old David, he may become unable to work and lose his income right when medical expenses are mounting. Likewise, many caregivers have given up their jobs to stay home to care for their loved ones.

When we sold the farm to the kids and moved into town, I got a job in a grain mill near our apartment so I could build up my Social Security. After about a year, it became clear that Emma wasn't safe alone. That's when I quit my job even though it meant I would get a lot less Social Security. Emma's safety is more important.

—Howard

Here are some suggestions for making your money go a bit further:

Pensions, insurances, and veteran's benefits:

- If individuals of wage-earning age are in danger of losing a job because of behavior issues that are unlike their past behaviors, or because of the inability to perform tasks they have been able to do in the past, insist upon an evaluation from a LBD-savvy physician *before* the job ends. If the physician diagnoses LBD, your loved one can retire with a disability pension.

- The Social Security Administration has added early onset Alzheimer's disease and related dementias to the fast track approval for Social Security Disability Insurance.[3] This allows someone younger than age 65 diagnosed with a degenerating dementia to obtain monthly pension benefits and Medicare much more quickly than the usual 2-year wait.

- Individuals older than 65 years of age are likely already on Medicare or have an insurance plan connected with Medicare. Check with their agent to see if they qualify for the low-income plan that many of these groups offer.

- There are several veteran's benefits worth checking out.[4] Spouses, widows, and dependent children also qualify for some of these services. Some of our country's most highly qualified dementia specialists work in Veteran Affairs (VA) hospitals and clinics, where care is free to low-income veterans. Often overlooked, the "aid and attendance benefit" helps with the cost of home care, assisted living, nursing homes, and medical expenses. This last benefit requires that the veteran be honorably discharged with at least 1 day served during wartime.

Medications and health care:

- Use generic drugs rather than brand name drugs whenever possible.

- Ask the doctor about less expensive choices for drugs. For instance, an over-the-counter drug such as ibuprofen (Advil) may be as effective as a more expensive prescription drug.

- Some drug companies will supply free drugs to people who meet their low-income requirements. Ask your pharmacist for more details.

- Some local agencies can help with medications, especially for a one-time event. Check with your local Area Agency on Aging.

> Exercise is much less expensive than drugs and slows down dementia, "better than any medication." The more your loved one exercises, the less medication he may need.

General finances:

- If your home is paid for, consider a reverse mortgage, which will allow you to live in your home and receive a monthly payment.

- If someone in the family cannot help with the caregiving but wants to assist in some other way, suggest that he or she help with monthly expenses.

- Many older people want to pass on as much of their savings to their children as they can and will therefore deny themselves the things they need and could afford if they used their savings. However, in most cases children would prefer that their parents use these funds to make their life more comfortable—and possibly longer—*now*. Adult children need to make this clear to their parents and free them to use their savings to make their final days more comfortable.

- If the caregiver is unable to handle the finances, find someone else to do it—another family member, a trusted friend, or a paid financial advisor, for instance. Finances handled correctly, bills paid on time, and other obligations met appropriately save money in the long run.

End-of-life expenses:

- Some research and/or medical centers will pay for funeral expenses if you donate your loved one's body to research. They do the research, cremate the body, and return the ashes to you within a few weeks.[5] In most cases, it is possible to designate a preferred type of research for the donation to benefit. However, a brain autopsy may not be one of the options. Therefore, you may have to make a choice.

- Cremation is much less expensive than burial. Unless someone in your family has a serious preference for burial, you can save thousands of dollars by choosing cremation.

- If you have medical bills left over after your loved one dies, most hospitals and clinics will offer a hefty discount when the bills are paid in full. If this is not possible, they will also work with you to set up affordable monthly payments.

14

End-of-Life Issues

Lewy body dementia (LBD) is a progressive disease. As one caregiver said, "The only way to beat Lewy is through death." Therefore, all LBD families must eventually face end-of-life issues. By that time, most caregivers will already have felt the loss of their loved ones as they once knew them. Now, the caregiver must face the loss of this person who has become as dependent on her as her children once were. Finally, a caregiver whose life has centered on the care of her loved one faces the loss of this job and other major changes once her loved one is gone.

How Long Can I Expect My Loved One to Live?

This is a common question and, like most things about LBD, there is no pat answer. The average life expectancy from diagnosis to death is 2 to 7 years, a bit shorter than the 3 to 9 years for Alzheimer's disease (AD). It is unusual for a person with LBD to live longer than 10 years past diagnosis, whereas someone with AD may live for another 20 years.

Alzheimer's is essentially a cognitive disorder, and a person is often in good physical health for most of the dementia journey. However, LBD is a many-faceted disorder, and a person with LBD will have other challenges that tend to decrease mobility, general health, and life expectancy.

In addition, when these other challenges are severe, they may cause equally severe episodes of LBD's unique fluctuations, with drastic dips in cognition and only small amounts of recovery that move a person toward the end more quickly than does the gradual slide of AD.

Anique's defining event was a surgery she had to have. Her mental condition plummeted afterward, and she died a few months later.

—*Jim*

The defining event does not have to be a surgery.

My Harry was really sick with colitis last year. He was never the same after that.

—*Nell*

Any illness adds stress that a person with LBD does not have the reserves to handle well. Other caregivers talk about drug sensitivities from which their loved ones never completely recover. Defining events may include more than one type of challenge. For instance, a severe drug sensitivity may occur due to the drugs used to treat a serious illness. Usually, there will be more than one defining event, with a decrease in cognitive functioning after each one until, finally, the end comes.

How Can I Prepare?

Once the financial and legal issues are in order, your main preparation will be learning what to expect and how to adjust from active to palliative caregiving, that is how to go from actively doing everything you can to help your loved one have a good quality of life to a more passive stage in which you help your loved one have a peaceful, painless end-of-life experience. This includes researching hospice options in your community well before you need this service.

> In the end stages of the LBD journey a caregiver's job changes from trying to extend her loved one's life to helping the loved one be comfortable and at peace.

How Do I Know the End Is Near?

Toward the end, your loved one will probably no longer be able to communicate directly, will be totally dependent on you or someone else for all of the personal care, and will be bedridden. He will likely sleep most of the time and will eat very little if anything at all.

When Peter started sleeping about 20 hours a day, the nurse told me this was normal for someone with end-stage dementia. And then, one day about 3 weeks after the nurse told me that, he just didn't wake up. I was so glad that he went so easily in the end.

—*Jenny*

Sleeping for long times, about 15 hours a day, is normal for someone with LBD, but when the time extends closer to 20 hours the end is probably near.

> The last time Anique was in the hospital, I stayed until she was asleep. Then I warned the staff that she always wanted to get up and go to the bathroom as soon as she woke up, and would fall down if she did (she had orthostatic hypotension). I got them to promise not to leave her alone, and then I went home to try to get some sleep myself. When I got back the next morning, I found that they had left her alone after all. The rails were up and they, not knowing about fluctuating cognition, had no idea that she'd be able to figure out how to get out—or that she'd physically be able to do so. She woke up, crawled to the foot of the bed where there were no rails and climbed out. Of course, she fell down after about three steps. A broken rib punctured her lung and she died 2 months later from various complications, including pneumonia.
>
> —*Jim*

Although your loved one may just slip away as Peter did, Anique's story is more common. People usually do not die from LBD; they die from complications, such as pneumonia. However, their dementia has usually progressed so far by then that the final period is a gentle wasting away with little pain or agitation. This was the case for Anique after her fall. Her cognition dipped sharply again, and during those last months she mostly slept, did not communicate except on the last evening, and did not appear agitated.

Toward the end, your loved one will become less willing to eat.[1] Swallowing has become an often-dangerous chore, and with the loss of the ability to taste and smell that accompanies LBD there is little reward. You can throw out the rule books about what he should and should not eat and feed him whatever he likes best. Expect him to eat only a spoonful or two; thus, every calorie counts.

Watch for "chipmunking"—the storage of food in one's cheeks. This is a prime cause of choking and aspiration, which can then lead to pneumonia.

Eventually, your loved one will probably refuse to eat or even drink. This is a normal part of the process. As the body begins to shut down, it no longer needs fuel. Some caregivers become concerned about their loved one starving and want to use feeding tubes. However, at this stage there is less discomfort connected to the "starving" than there is in trying to digest food that is no longer needed.

Although your loved one may not have much cognitive ability left, he can feel emotions. Moreover, although he may no longer communicate, he probably can hear and may still be able to comprehend at least some of what he hears. Give him a lot of touching and affection, but be careful about what you say, especially when you and another person are talking near your loved one's bedside. Remember that the LBD confusion is still present. Your loved one may overhear a perfectly innocent statement, turn it into something scary, and become agitated.

He can also feel pain, and change will continue to be stressful, especially when he can no longer even begin to reason about why you or others are treating him this way. Feeding tubes are both painful and uncomfortable. Sudden trips to the emergency room to treat dehydration or infections can be more stressful than they are worth. At this point, you need to evaluate everything you do by how it affects your loved one's comfort rather than by how it prolongs his life.

Be very gentle when you touch your loved one. His skin will become quite delicate and sensitive. It is likely that he will lose the ability to move himself, so do not let him lie in one position for too long or his skin will break down, resulting in painful pressure sores that can become infected.

Although the *good times* of fluctuating cognition will become rare, caregivers tell many poignant stories of windows of awareness that occur near the end. Jim told earlier about how Anique was able to recognize him and differentiate between their two daughters the evening before she died. However, the following anecdote is one of our favorites:

> It used to be that when I felt discouraged, I'd talk it over with Jerry, my husband and best friend of over 40 years. He'd listen and give me a hug and I'd feel better. But the Jerry who had been my rock in so many storms was gone, and there was just this shell of a man there on the bed. One day, not long after my dear friend Julie died, I was feeling particularly down and really needed at least the memory of Jerry's comforting. So, I sent the caregiver away, sat by Jerry's bed, and

laid my head against his arm. I told him my problems; tears came and I let them fall. I didn't expect anything from Jerry, but it felt good just being there with him. And then I felt something touch my hair. My dear husband, who hadn't talked in months, who usually didn't even recognize me, was slowly and awkwardly trying to pat my head. A month later, I lost Jerry too, but I'll always remember that special moment we had close to the end.

—Camille

Other caregivers tell of how their loved one waited for one last member of the family to arrive before they let go of life.

Darla had been going downhill for a long time when the staff warned me she'd only last a few days more. She seldom responded even to me and didn't seem to know when others were in the room at all. But I called the kids anyway. I knew they'd want to give their mother a final goodbye. The two girls were able to get here right away, but our son, Brandon, lives several states away. And then there was a storm and the planes were grounded, and it took him an extra 2 days to make it. When I told Darla that Brandon was coming and why he wasn't there yet, she didn't seem to respond. But when Brandon finally came in and gave his mother a kiss, she sighed and within an hour she was gone.

—John

You may think your loved one is not capable of knowing what is going on or that they are not able to recognize family members anymore, but do not count on that. Remember, hearing and comprehension last long after the ability to communicate has gone. So, do encourage the family to come and say goodbye, and do let your loved one know if someone has been delayed, as Brandon was. If someone important cannot come at all, consider a final phone call.

Even after there appears to be little cognition left, a person with LBD may have a short period of awareness in which you can say your goodbyes. Persons who have lost the ability to communicate may also be more aware than they appear.

What About Hospice?

Hospice provides end-of-life medical, psychological, and spiritual support. Its goal is to control pain and other symptoms so that your loved one can remain as alert and comfortable as possible. Hospice programs also provide services to support their patients' families.[2]

Hospice is a service provided by various profit and not-for-profit companies. A person who qualifies goes "on hospice" and, while in the program, stays "in service," according to hospice syntax.

Who Is Eligible for Hospice?

Before hospice services can begin, a physician must certify that a person has a life expectancy of 6 months *or* has dementia and *all* of the following:

- Requires assistance with dressing, walking, and bathing;
- Has urinary and fecal incontinence; and
- Cannot speak or have a meaningful conversation.

Your loved one may already have other complications, such as recurrent infections, pneumonia, or other LBD-related problems that support the life expectancy criteria, even if he is not completely helpless.

To receive hospice services, the family must agree to use only palliative medications, that is, those that provide only pain relief and comfort. Many of the medications prescribed for LBD do improve comfort, and thus this requirement may not be an issue. However, other medications, such as those for a heart problem, would likely be considered life saving rather than palliative and would have to be dropped.[3]

Why Some Families Do Not Use Hospice Fully

Misunderstanding the Criteria

Some families believe that hospice is only for people who are actively dying, that hospice services are needed only for the last few weeks or days of life, when a person is quite debilitated. It is important to remember that the guidelines clearly allow for a 6-month life expectancy. A person with a degenerative disease such as Lewy body dementia is a much different person 6 months prior to his death than he is a few weeks prior. He likely still has the ability to enjoy life and to communicate. He probably still has occasional *good times* that last longer than just a few minutes. However, the caregiving will be more difficult, and the services that hospice provides would be very useful.

The Belief That Hospice Means Giving Up

Most families have been doing battle against this disease for years, making every effort to prolong and enhance their loved ones' lives. Deciding to use hospice care requires a change of goals that some find difficult to make. However, recognizing that the disease has progressed to the stage where comfort is more important than extending life is not giving up; it is an acceptance of your loved one's true needs and a willingness to put those first. Prolonging life may still be the family's need, but is it their loved one's need? Often the best gift, and perhaps the most difficult, is permission to let go. One caregiver put it this way: "I do the best I can to make his dying easier while, with all my heart, I wish he could continue to live."

Unwillingness to Admit That the End Is Near

Not only families but loved ones as well may feel this way and resist hospice. Reframing hospice as a valuable assistance and the end-of-life requirement as a challenge to beat can help.

> My grandmother had mild LBD along with a serious heart problem. She got angry when her doctor suggested hospice. She complained, "The doctor told me I had to die in 6 months if I accepted hospice care. Well, I'm not ready to die!" I assured her that this was only an estimate, not a requirement, and so she agreed to accept. Grandma lived on hospice for 18 months. We were so glad for this service. It gave Mom some much-needed help and Grandma liked all the extra attention. We especially liked the caring attitude of all the workers.
>
> —*Lee*

As Lee told her grandmother, the 6-month requirement is only an estimate. They will not drop your loved one from their service if he lives longer than 6 months—unless, of course, he appears to be getting better and no longer fits the criteria. Some people have been on hospice for as long as 4 years.

Fear That Medications Will Be Stopped

It is true that, by definition, hospice care is palliative. However, some programs consider those drugs used for dementia or acting out to be palliative, because they make life more comfortable. Others may not, and may require that at least the cognition drugs be stopped. Because this varies from program to program, be sure to inquire about your loved one's specific medications when you interview prospective hospices.

Physician Hesitation

Some physicians are hesitant to recommend hospice until a person is actively dying. One roadblock is the 6-month test. Some physicians may state that they cannot say how a particular individual will fare. A better suggestion is for physician to ask himself or herself, "Would I be surprised if this patient was dead within 6 months?" If the answer is "no," then this patient is a candidate for hospice care.[4]

How Can I Find a Hospice Service?

There are many hospice service providers in every community. The problem is generally not one of finding a service, but of finding the right one. For example, in the metropolitan Phoenix area there are more than 200 hospice groups. Some accept patients with dementia, and some do not. Of those that accept patients with dementia, some have staff trained to work with patients with dementia, and some do not. Of those who are trained to work with dementia, some have been trained about the differences between AD and LBD, and some have not. It is the same in most large communities.

Interview prospective hospice programs just as you would adult day care or residential programs. Start by asking some general questions about what services they provide, who provides them, and where. Then, ask some LBD-specific questions:

- How familiar are you with the sensitivity of patients with LBD to certain medications, including many strong pain drugs?

- Which of my loved one's medications are considered palliative and which, if any, are not? What will happen about those that are not?

- What will happen if my loved one becomes very ill and needs to be hospitalized?

- What do you know about LBD and its fluctuations, including *showtime*?

Who Pays for Hospice?

For people who are eligible for Medicare, hospice is free. It is included in all Medicare-based insurance plans and is governed by Medicare regulations. Some insurances also cover hospice. If a patient does not qualify for Medicare and has no insurance that covers hospice, then other arrangements can be made, depending on the hospice group the family chooses.

What Does a Hospice Provide?

Although this will vary slightly with the hospice group you choose, all are required by Medicare to offer the following services:

- *Home health aides:* These individuals help with bathing and other personal care services several times a week. This service alone can sometimes mean the difference between being able to keep your loved one home and having to place him in a residential facility.

- *Nurses:* A nurse can make house calls and perform regular checks on your loved one's condition. Family caregivers who have bundled up their loved ones, complete with wheelchair or walker, struggled to get them in and out of the car, then sat in a waiting room far too long to be seen for much too short a time can appreciate a nurse who makes house calls.

- *Volunteers:* Volunteers visit regularly and can stay with the patient while the caregiver can take some time for herself. As your loved one's dementia increases, visitors just for him usually decrease. Volunteers are wonderful. They are there as your loved one's personal visitors. They have the time to sit and listen. The stories everyone else has heard repeatedly are new and interesting to the volunteer. Alternatively, if your loved one is beyond visiting and storytelling, volunteers know how to be a comfortable presence.

- *Social workers and chaplains:* These trained individuals offer emotional and spiritual support.

My first experience with hospice was while taking care of my sister, Lucille. She was on hospice, and they took wonderful care of her. But they told me "There are two of you in this family. We're here for you, too." Thousands of miles away from my friends and stuck in my sister's tiny apartment, I did not have anyone to vent to, and I was not getting enough exercise. When I shared my concerns with the hospice social worker, she invited me to go walking with her once a week. We both got some exercise while she listened to my gripes. I went home feeling much more able to care for my sister with the patience she deserved. I was so impressed by the way hospice helped both my sister and me that I eventually became a hospice volunteer.

- *Medical equipment:* Certain medical equipment will help make your loved one more comfortable. For example, a hospital bed makes it a great deal easier to care for a bedridden person but is far too expensive for the average family. Most hospice services have loaner beds as well as other equipment, such as bedside commodes and wheelchairs.

- *Palliative drugs:* Drugs used to decrease pain or agitation will be paid for by the hospice service. These may or may not include acting-out drugs, such as quetiapine (Seroquel), but do include opiates and other strong pain medications. Be sure your hospice nurse is aware that LBD makes a person very sensitive to these drugs.

- *Respite care in a residential facility:* Although most hospice service is provided in the home, the hospice service probably also has a residential facility where loved ones can go if:

  - They become ill and need round-the-clock nursing. Hospice services always prefer that their patients enter their respite facilities instead of a hospital whenever possible.

  - The family caregiver needs a more than a few hours off. She can go for several days and know that her loved one is safe and well cared for.

- *Grief counseling:* This can start prior to your loved one's death and can continue for months afterward. Chaplains and social workers offer individual and group grief counseling for family members during a rough time. Take advantage of this service when the time comes, because it will help you deal with the many changes you must face.

When Should We Start Hospice?

The bottom-line answer to this question is "As soon as you can possibly qualify." One of the mistakes LBD caregivers often make is that they do not start hospice soon enough. The advantages of obtaining hospice care as soon as your loved one qualifies are huge. All the services that hospice provides will lighten your load and may make it possible for you to keep your loved one at home until the end.

People on hospice tend to live longer than they would without this service. The peaceful and stress-free existence encouraged by hospice services, the good nursing, and all the attention a person under hospice care gets have a positive and life-extending effect. After all, decreasing stress is one of the most important things you can do to help your loved one function at his fullest. Therefore, investigate hospice well before you need it, be aware of just what is required to qualify, and apply as soon as you think your loved one may be eligible.

What Happens if My Loved One Gets Better?

To stay on hospice, a person's condition must continue to degenerate. Medicare requires that someone whose physical condition appears to be improving be dropped from hospice service until a physician has again certified that he qualifies. The same is true if a person with dementia appears to have become less helpless. And therein lies a possible problem for the LBD family.

> We were so pleased when we got Larry on hospice. He was bedridden and didn't have very many *good times* any more— never more than a few minutes long. Then, after Larry had only been in the program a few months, the social worker came to visit and Larry did a *showtime* recovery act. He even talked with the social worker—and he hadn't talked in weeks. The social worker reported Larry's "improved" condition and the staff took him off their service. They said he didn't qualify anymore.
>
> —*Judy*

This is a much too common refrain among LBD caregivers. If your hospice staff are not educated about fluctuating cognition and *showtime*, your family could face the same issues. Start by asking questions about LBD during your interview, and continue by making sure that any of the staff, from the hospice physician to the aides, know about *showtime*.

Hospice

- Lightens your workload and provides medical support to your loved one,

- Provides emotional and spiritual support to both of you,

- May actually help your loved one to live longer,

- Often allows him to live out his final days at home, and

- Helps you with your grief after he is gone.

This end-of-life period is usually a time of waiting for the caregiver. Hope for more time has changed to hope for a peaceful end. It is easy to feel emotional, and there is certainly nothing wrong with that. However, save your crying for when you are not with your loved one—or for later. What he one needs now is your calm presence, your caring, and your acceptance.

15

How Do I Take Care of Myself?

You are the most important person in your loved one's life. You are his lifeline, his connection to continuity, and the person who knows him best. Therefore, caring for yourself is a key part of being a caregiver—and one that often gets neglected. This should come as no surprise; caregiving is usually a job taken on out of love for the person, not a desire for the job itself—a job the caregiver knew little about before being forced to learn.

> I didn't sign on for this. It was not the way I planned to spend my retirement years. But I love my husband and I want to be here for him.
>
> —*Jenny*

> "Caregivers are people who, once the need is there, step up and do the job with love and to the best of their ability."
>
> —*Anonymous*

Jim knew very little about caregiving before Lewy body dementia (LBD) entered his life. As he learned what he was facing, he felt overwhelmed. He could afford to hire help, and he did, but as Anique's condition degenerated even that was not enough, and eventually he had to place her in a residential facility.

Jenny's unwanted responsibility made her job more isolating because the person she used to depend on for support was no longer able to provide it.

More than anything, I missed the partner I used to have. Peter
was my best friend. We did everything together. But after he got
so bad, I had to make the decisions, and telling him my troubles
just made him upset. He wasn't able to support me anymore.

—*Jenny*

Jenny needed to develop a new support system and was fortunate
to find a local caregivers support group.

My support group has been my lifeline. They've told me where
to find a good lawyer, given me many caregiving tips, been there
when I needed a shoulder to cry on, and so much more.

—*Jenny*

Marie is part of the "sandwich generation," those caring for elderly
parents or, in her case, a dementia-impaired spouse and children as well.

I'm the family breadwinner now that David had to quit his job
because of the problems his dementia was causing. I feel pulled
in so many different ways! I'm a part-time interior decorator,
and I love my job but it's demanding. Even when I didn't have
David to worry about, it took much of my energy. And then
there are the children. I want them to have a good childhood,
but sometimes I feel like I don't have enough energy to be there
for them. David does what he can, but I never know when he'll
have a bad day. I don't like to leave them alone with him—he
gets so mad over nothing.

—*Marie*

Marie is just starting the LBD journey. One of the biggest mistakes
family caregivers make is to try to do it all themselves. Marie needs to
learn now, early in her journey, to ask for help—and to accept it when
it is offered. This can be a great lifesaver, especially later, when the job
gets even more difficult.

Karl's LBD has been gradually getting worse over the last
4 years, but I thought I was managing—barely. I had my groceries and even our medicines delivered. The only time I'd get
out of the house was to take Karl to a doctor's appointment. I
knew I wasn't taking very good care of myself, but there just

didn't seem to be enough time or energy left for me once I'd done everything I needed to do for Karl.

Then I fell, and everything changed. I have diabetes, and I guess I let my blood sugar get too high, and I fainted. I crawled over to the phone and called 911. I didn't know who else to call. I don't have any friends anymore, what with not being able to leave Karl alone and him getting so obnoxious when I have visitors—I guess he's jealous. Anyway, the paramedics took us both to the hospital. The doctor said I'd have to stay until my diabetes was stabilized, and they kept Karl overnight. I called my daughter, Janey. She flew in and took Karl back to our house and stayed with him until I could come home. But she has a job and a family, so she couldn't stay long. Before she left, she did arrange for a caregiver to come in three times a week to help me with Karl. I should have done that a long time ago.

—*Paula*

Paula's story is a good example of how not to take care of your loved one. She was so intent on taking care of her husband that she did not take care of her own health. She did not take any time for herself. She let her friendships lapse and was not even going out for groceries, let alone church or other personal activities. She was trying to do an around-the-clock job without help, and it was wearing her out. Finally, her body rebelled.

When we fly, the flight attendant warns us that if the plane loses pressure, we need to put on our air mask before we help anyone else. The heart pumps blood to itself before it pumps blood to the rest of the body. Likewise, caregivers must be just as diligent about taking care of themselves so that they can care for their loved ones. This includes maintaining good emotional and spiritual health so that they can provide a calm environment for their loved ones. If a caregiver is distressed in any way—sick, tired, frustrated, whatever—her loved one will reflect that with acting-out behavior that will likely distress her—and him—even more.

Care for the Family Caregiver[1] is a booklet that covers this subject very thoroughly. You can download it free from the Internet or order it from the National Alliance for Caregiving.[2] However, here are some ways to care for your body and spirit to get you started.

Take Care of Your Health

- *Make your doctor's appointments and keep them.* With all the time spent taking your loved one to the doctor, getting prescriptions and such, you may not feel up to more medical scenarios. However, if you neglect your own health you could end up like Paula, unable to care for your loved one and with no one to call in an emergency. See your dentist regularly too, because oral health is closely associated with overall well-being.

- *Exercise.* Exercise is as important for the caregiver because it is for her loved one. "I don't have the time or energy" is not a good excuse. Even if you must get up earlier in the morning, the benefits of a 15-minute—or preferably longer—walk are worth it. Use a stationary bicycle or do aerobics if it is difficult to get out of the house. You will feel energized and better able to face your day. If you can find someone who will exercise with you, that is even better.

- *Eat healthy.* It is so easy to live on fast food and snacks, especially when fixing separate meals for your loved one and yourself. Like exercise, your nutritional health is as important as your loved one's. For more energy, add plenty of fresh vegetables to your diet and decrease the amount of starch and sugar.

Do Not Try to Do It All Yourself

- *Ask for help.* Caregivers say repeatedly that this was the most difficult thing to learn to do. However, not asking for help leads to burnout. Start looking for helping agencies before you need them, and use their services when you do need them.

- *Hire a respite caregiver occasionally.* Even if your budget is limited, this is a necessity, not a luxury. Plan to do something for yourself while the helper is there. After the first time or so, *do not* stay with your loved one while the helper is there. Until you are comfortable leaving them alone, go into another part of the house and work on a craft project, take a nap, or watch a favorite TV program. After the first time or two, you should be able to leave them alone. Go out. Do something for yourself. Go get your hair or nails done. Call a friend and go out to lunch or to a movie.

- *Accept help from other family members and close friends.* Do not forget, this is their loved one too, and they will probably be happy to help.

My son, Jonathan, always lets me know when he's going to visit Mom so I can make arrangements to go out and get my hair done or have lunch with a friend. I so appreciate his help and Mom loves having his full attention.

—Marion, daughter of Clara

Drop-in friends and relatives who volunteer to help are wonderful, and you can still go out, but planning as Jonathan and Marion do gives the caregiver a chance to make appointments and do things she might otherwise not be able to do.

- *Accept funds from family members who want to help but cannot do so physically.* Use this money to hire respite caregivers, someone to provide a few hours a week of regular home health care or even overnight. Family members and friends who want to help but cannot assist physically should suggest this to the family caregiver. Family caregivers should speak up and ask for needed financial help. Helping financially is an important way of being a part of a loved one's care.

- *Have a list of things people can do to help.* Often, friends or relatives will ask what they can do. The easiest—and the least helpful—answer is to tell them "I don't know." If you have not thought about it, you probably *do not* know. So take some time to make a list of tasks that people could do to help: shopping, doing dishes, vacuuming, sitting with your loved one for an hour, walking with you, anything. Just brainstorm. You will be surprised at what you can come up with. Then when someone asks, get out your list.

Get Enough Sleep

When your loved one has active dreams or wanders at night, or has other issues that keep you up or keep you from sleeping soundly, it is easy to become tired and run down.

- Caregivers suggest power naps. Take a 15-minute nap while your loved one is sleeping.
- Use the time to nap when a home health care worker, friend, or family member is there.

These refreshing naps will make the rest of the day go better and your tasks seem easier.

Maintain Your Personal Support System

- *Keep in touch with your friends.* It is worth the effort.

I used to have a couple of very good friends. We'd meet once in awhile to have lunch and giggle and act like girls. It was fun, and I always came home feeling better. But that's gone now. Oh, they call once in awhile, but I never call them anymore. There's so much to do here I feel guilty taking time for myself. If I call when Jake's awake, he gets jealous. Heaven help me if they come to visit! The last time one of my friends came to visit, he just asked outright when she was going to go home. I was grateful he didn't try to shove her out the door!

Anyway, my friends and I don't seem to have much to talk about anymore. Our lives are so different now. Oh, they try to understand but it's just not the same—and not worth the bother. I'm so glad I found this online support group. I can even go online in the middle of the night, like after Jake wakes me up with a bad dream. Once I get him settled and back to sleep, I'm usually wide awake! But now, I get on the computer and see what's happening in the group and write something myself. The people there understand. They've been where I am. I love the support I get!

—Norma

Jake's behavior is very common—a person with advanced LBD seldom likes to share their loved one's attention. Do not let such behavior stop you from maintaining contact with old friends. Talk on the phone when your loved one is asleep. Meet them away from your loved one—in another room while he is sleeping, for instance—or, even better, find someone to sit with your loved one while you go out with them for an hour or so.

Sadly, Norma's observation that she and her friends seem to have little in common anymore is often true. Caregiving takes up one's whole life, and things that used to be important fall by the wayside. That is where caregiver support groups come in.

- *Support group:* Dementia caregivers need a place where they can vent, share ideas, and ask questions, where others understand because they have the same issues. A support group provides such a forum.

Thank goodness I have my support group. When my health aide insisted that I try going, I wasn't sure I should leave Emma that long. But I come back feeling so much better and more able to cope. We can relate. I hate to bore my friends, and besides, they don't really understand. My family supports me, but they don't understand either. You can't if you haven't lived it.

—Howard

Howard can vent and his group knows he is simply frustrated; he does not want out. He can ask "How do you handle this?" and get answers from others who have had the same problem. He can make *dark jokes* about his situation and his group members are not shocked; they laugh with him. He goes home feeling better about himself and his situation.

- *Online groups:* If you have a computer, consider joining an online LBD caregiver's support group. There are several listed on the Lewy Body Dementia Association (LBDA) Web site. The beauty of an online group is that, like Norma, you can be there at any time—three o'clock in the morning, six o'clock at night, or whenever you can have a few minutes free.

I found an online LBD caregivers group a couple of years before Anique died. There weren't many men in it, or if they were, they were just lurking—that's reading, but not posting. That's all I did at first too. But then I had a problem I didn't know how to solve. Anique could no longer go to the bathroom by herself. What was I to do when we were out and she needed to go? I took this to my group. "Maybe we should just stop going out," I told them. I was amazed at how many answered and the amount of understanding and caring support I got. "No, no," they all insisted. They told me about a law that allows a person of the opposite sex to go into a public bathroom to assist a handicapped person. "Don't let this stop you from taking your wife out," they said. It was a great feeling to know that there were people like me out there willing to help and share their own experiences. Some of those people are still my friends today.

—Jim

Jim is still a moderator of that group. He makes a special effort to welcome new men when they show up with a question. There are a few more men in the online groups today than there were 10 years ago, but Jim says that the gender differences are not important. The caregiving issues are the same.

- *Local groups:* Finding a local group that works for an LBD caregiver may not be as easy as finding an online group.
  - If you are fortunate, your local community will have an LBDA-sponsored caregiver's support group. Visit the LBDA Web site (www.lbda.org) and click on the "Find Support" tab. If there is not an LBDA group in your area, and you would like to start one, contact the LBDA. No formal education is required, and the LBDA provides training and support.
  - The Alzheimer's Association and various Parkinson's organizations sponsor caregiver groups in most areas. Keep in mind that these groups may not cover all the problems that are unique to LBD. Although AD groups provide great support for dementia problems, the members may not be able to relate to LBD symptoms such as hallucinations and active dreams. PD groups are great for movement issues; however, because patients often attend these groups with their caregivers, the dementia symptoms and behavior management issues tend to be avoided. If a group cannot support a caregiver adequately, it may increase her sense of isolation.
  - Contact the local Area Agency on Aging for further information on other local caregiver groups.

- ○ Prior to attending a group, contact the group facilitator and ask the following questions to see whether the group is a good fit:
    - Are you familiar with Lewy body dementia and its two types?
    - Do any members of your group have loved ones with LBD? (Try to find a group with at least two other LBD caregivers.)
    - Are your groups for caregivers only, or are the loved ones invited? (This is a caregiver choice, but most LBD caregivers prefer the freedom of discussing dementia and acting-out issues without their loved one present.)
    - Is there an accompanying respite program so that I can bring my loved one and leave him in a safe place while I attend the group? (If finding a sitter is an issue, this may be quite important.)

Take Breaks

- *Give yourself time-outs.* When something stressful occurs, take a 5-minute time-out. Step out onto the back porch. Go hide out in the bathroom. Sneak into a closet, if you must, then:
    - ○ Take some deep breaths, think some pleasant thoughts, and relax;
    - ○ Look for a way to laugh at the stress-producing situation; or
    - ○ Think of at least one thing to be grateful for this minute.

It is amazing how just 5 short minutes and a change of perspective can reduce stress.

- *Take regular respite times.* Do not neglect to take some time just for you. This means more than just long enough to do some shopping and hurry back. Your loved one, who deals poorly with change and probably has fears of abandonment, may resist. He may act frightened, cry, or act out when you leave for any length of time. Do not let this stop you. Staying will only lead to more burnout. You need that time away so that you can give your loved one better care when you return.

The best way to plan respites is to start early in the LBD journey, while your loved one still has the ability to see your needs and the security to know you will be returning, probably in a much better mood.

As a nurse, I knew about the burnout that can happen when caregivers do not take time for themselves. So when I agreed to go live with my sister, Lucille, and care for her during her final months, I did so with the understanding that she would hire a respite caregiver for my occasional days off. She agreed, and even very late in her illness, when she really did not want me to go, she accepted it as a part of our routine. Of course, one reason this worked was that we had a very good respite caregiver. I also called a few times while I was gone so Lucille would know I had not forgotten her—and so I would know everything was all right at home.

Once your loved one is on hospice, respite is much easier to find. Volunteers and staff will stay with your loved one several hours a week. For longer periods, there is usually a residential respite facility where you can feel very safe leaving him for several days.

- *Tag team.* If there are two caregivers in the family, tag-teaming works wonderfully.

My mother-in-law lived with us for years. She had LBD, but at first, it was hardly noticeable, and we all did fine. Then her dementia got worse, and some of her acting-out behaviors were hard for me to deal with. That's when my husband and I learned to tag-team. When whatever Mom was doing got to me so much that I just wanted to scream, Randall would tell me, "I'll watch her for awhile." I'd go give myself a time-out and calm down. Then there were the times when it was the other way around.

—*Catherine*

Consider some code words to use so your partner knows you need a break.

Adult day care was another great help for us. We learned to use this especially when both of us were feeling frazzled. And Mom loved it. The people there were really good to her.

—*Catherine*

- *Adult day care.* This is not just for a caregiver who is working or needs to run errands. It is also there to give a frustrated caregiver a break—or to prevent the frustration in the first place. Visits can be a daily event for a few hours, or once a week, or whatever fits your family needs.

Maintain Your Emotional Health

- *Recognize your feelings.* We have little control over what we feel but, unlike our damaged loved ones, we do have control over how we choose to express our feelings, and that can often change the way we feel.

Anger is a good example. Most caregivers will have periods when they feel angry. It is all too easy to be upset with your loved one and at the frustrating things he does. Even if you do not say anything, he will perceive this anger as abandonment, a major fear of any helpless person—and his anger-causing behavior will likely increase. Direct your feelings at the disease instead. After all, your loved one also has his own anger issues with LBD. United against a common enemy, you will have a common bond. He will feel closer to you instead of abandoned, and his acting-out behaviors will likely decrease.

- *Do not go on guilt trips.* Guilt trips never go anywhere helpful. They just pull you down. Guilt is a way of trying to control something that is uncontrollable. Let it go. No matter what has happened, guilt will only immobilize you. It does not let you move forward.
  - It is not wrong to leave your loved one with someone while you go enjoy yourself for awhile.
  - It is not wrong to ask for help.
  - It is not wrong to feel trapped in a job you did not ask for.
  - It is not wrong to feel angry.
  - It is not wrong to. . . . Just let it all go.

- *Be alert for signs of depression.* This is a lurking danger for LBD caregivers. When your loved one has smeared feces all over the wall, the bank account is overdrawn because no one took the time to balance the checkbook, and your arthritic back hurts, depression may seem unavoidable. However, it is possible to fight it, and if you do, these problems will all seem less overwhelming.

Fight depression by using all of the caregiving suggestions mentioned so far:

- Having a support group, even if it is a few friends you can call on whenever you feel down—or excited.
- Maintaining your health by making and keeping doctor's appointments, eating a healthy diet, and maintaining a regular exercise routine.
- Taking regular "me" times, including occasional longer respite periods.
- Getting adequate sleep, even if it is via "power naps."
- Being willing to ask for help and accepting it when offered.
- Making an effort to see the positives and looking for ways to feel grateful.

If all else fails, talk to your doctor about medication. What you likely have is called *situational depression*. It can often be decreased significantly by the suggestions mentioned earlier, but if you still feel down some of the same drugs recommended for your loved one may help you.

You Do Not Have to Be Alone

When the person who used to be your companion, partner, and helpmate is now a shell of his former self, unable to communicate much, and dependent on you for his care, it is easy feel alone. You do not have to be. Caregiving works best when it is a team effort.

- Start this journey by surrounding yourself with trustworthy LBD-savvy professionals. Once your professional team is in place, relax and let the team members take care of their jobs while you do yours: being the expert on your loved one's own special responses to this always-unique disease.

- Make use of the telephone and computer to maintain contact with support systems—family, friends, and a caregiver support group.

- Use some of the resources in this book and others, or information gathered online, to find help and respite care—and then use it.

Fill your life with people who can and will provide support. The effort is well worth the trouble—not only to you but also to your loved one, who will have a healthier and happier caregiver. Finally, do not forget that one of those supportive people must be you. Even with helpful friends and family, it will still be up to you to take care of the caregiver.

Moving On

Once your loved one has completed his LBD journey, there will be a time when you must obtain death certificates, notify various people and organizations of your loved one's death, and perform a multitude of related tasks. Once those are done, you will go from a life that has been overburdened with responsibilities to feeling as though you have far too little to do. In addition, you will go from a time filled with caring to a time filled with loss: the loss of your loved one, of a job that had come to define who you were, and of friends you had no time for before but now need.

Allow yourself to cry, and find someone to cry with. Crying is most helpful if done with someone. If you have lost touch with your friends during your LBD journey, the hospice grief groups mentioned earlier can be a great help, as can a social worker and chaplain. If you have a home church, talk to your pastor.

Do not let embarrassment about not maintaining contact when you were so involved with your loved one stop you from reaching out now to friends who have given up and disappeared. They will probably understand and be glad to resume the friendship. If you belong to a local caregivers group, do not drop out right away. You still need their support—and others need your experience. If you belong to an online group, be sure to let them know what has happened. You will be amazed at the support they can give you, too.

Do not be surprised, or even feel guilty, to realize that you have already grieved and are actually ready to move on surprisingly soon. The length of your grieving time is NOT a measure of your love. When, like Camille's Jerry, your loved one's personality is nearly gone, leaving only a helpless shell with little quality of life, it is normal for you to start grieving for the person you once knew. Many LBD caregivers say that by the time their loved one dies they have finished much of their grieving for the person they used to know. Now they must grieve only for that dependent person who was left.

You may think your grieving is done one day and feel devastated the next. You will likely fluctuate among depression, guilt, anger, and acceptance.[3] This is all part of the grieving process. When you notice that you are feeling angry more than guilty or depressed, you are well on the way toward acceptance—and moving on. Just as depression and guilt can immobilize, anger can motivate. Jim used his anger to move on when he helped start the LBDA. Other caregivers find something very different to put their energy into.

> I always wanted to travel, but Ben was happier just puttering around at home. And then, of course, after he developed dementia, we couldn't travel. It was just too difficult. Now that I'm alone, I've started traveling. First, I just went to visit my son for a week. And then my daughter and I took a lovely trip to visit her first grandchild. And now, I'm planning a cruise with some of the women from my online support group. I haven't forgotten Ben—how could I do that? But I am moving on and feeling ever so much better now that I'm doing something I've always wanted to do.
>
> —*Dora*

The main thing is to do something. Anything. It will do your loved one no good if you do not enjoy the life you have. You are alive. Live.

Glossary

Although many of these terms do not appear in the text of this book, you may come across them as you read other materials and talk to professionals.

NOTE: Italicized words within definitions are also shown in the glossary. Italicized words in parentheses after the definition refer to related subjects. For instance, the words after the definition for Aricept include other dementia drugs.

Acetylcholine (ACh): A key chemical in neurons (nerve cells) that acts as a neurotransmitter and carries information between two nerve cells.

Acetylcholinesterase inhibitor (AChEI): Medication that inhibits the enzymes that convert *acetylcholine* into other chemicals, thus increasing the level of acetylcholine in the brain. These drugs can decrease confusion, *cognitive fluctuations*, and other LBD symptoms, such as *agitation* and *hallucinations*, but often have severe gastrointestinal side effects. *(Aricept, Exelon, Razadyne)*

Activities of daily living (ADLs): Personal care activities necessary for everyday living, such as eating, bathing, grooming, dressing, mobility, and toileting. A person's amount of dementia is sometimes measured by these limitations.

Adult day care: A place where adults living at home can go during the day for activities, socializing, education, physical therapy, and health care. They provide participants opportunities to interact with others and caregivers time for respite.

Adverse drug reaction: An unexpected, unwanted, or dangerous reaction to a drug, and usually the opposite of the usual effect. The onset of the adverse reaction may be sudden or may develop over time. Also termed "adverse effect" or "adverse event."

Agitation: Excessive motor activity associated with a feeling of inner tension manifesting as verbal and physical aggression and active resistance to care. This can be seen as pacing, fidgeting, hand wringing, pulling of clothes, and the inability to sit still.

Agnosia (ag-NOH-zee-uh): The inability to recognize and identify objects or persons despite having knowledge of the characteristics of those objects or persons. People with agnosia may retain their cognitive abilities in other areas.

Akathisia (ak-uh-THIZH-uh): A movement disorder characterized by a feeling of inner restlessness and a compelling need to be in constant motion, often manifested through fidgeting.

Akinesia (ey-ki-NEE-zhuh): The loss of voluntary movement or impairment of movement. Akinesia is a term used in neurology to denote the absence of movement.

Alpha-synuclein: One in a family of structurally related proteins that are prominently expressed in the central nervous system.

Alzheimer's disease: A progressive neurodegenerative disease of the brain.

Ambien: The trade name for **zolpidem tartrate** (zole-puh-dem tar-trate), a medication used to treat patients with insomnia.

Ambulatory: Able to ambulate or walk about; not bedridden or hospitalized.

Ambulatory care: Medical care including diagnosis, observation, treatment, and rehabilitation that is provided on an outpatient basis to individuals who are able to ambulate or walk about.

Amnesia: Forgetfulness for details of recent events, conversations, and upcoming appointments.

Amyloid (AM-uh-loid): Any of several complex proteins that can be deposited in tissues, including organ-specific areas such as the central nervous system, as in Alzheimer's, Parkinson's, Huntington's, and Lewy body disease.

Amyloid precursor protein (APP): A gene that when mutated causes an abnormal form of the amyloid protein to be produced.

Antianxiety drug: Medication used to decrease agitation, nervousness, anxiety, and tension. Also called tranquilizers. It often causes severe side effects with LBD patients. (*anxiety*, Atarax, *Klonopin*, Valium)

Anticholinergic effect: A chemical effect that interferes with or lessens memory and thinking functions and may increase sleepiness and risks of imbalance or falling.

Anticonvulsive drug: Medication that reduces excessive nerve signals in the brain and restores the normal balance of nerve activity. These drugs may also be used to treat *depression* or *restless legs syndrome*. (*Neurontin, Tegretol*)

Antidepressant drug: Medication used to reduce depression. (*Celexa, Desyrel, Paxil, Prozac, selective serotonin reuptake inhibitors, Zoloft*)

Antihistamine: A medication commonly used in over-the-counter cold and allergy products. It can have *anticholinergic effects*.

Antipsychotic drug: Medication used to relieve *hallucinations, delusions, agitation*, and panic attacks. Also called *neuroleptic drug*. **Traditional antipsychotics** block neurotransmitter receptors, thus preventing nerves from being activated. Up to 50% of LBD patients have severe *neuroleptic sensitivity (Haldol)*. **Atypical antipsychotics** use a different action than traditional antipsychotics and are therefore usually, but not always, safer for LBD patients. (*Seroquel, Risperdal, Zyprexa*)

Anxiety: An abnormal and overwhelming sense of apprehension and fear, often marked by sweating, tension, and increased pulse, that affects everyday functioning.

Apathy: A lack of motivation to initiate conversations or perform activities.

Aphasia (uh-FEY-zhuh): The deterioration of language function. It is a severe form of dysphasia.

Aricept (AR-uh-sept): The trade name for **donepezil hydrochloride** (do-NEP-uh-zil HI-dro-klor-ide), an *acetylcholinesterase inhibitor* used to treat mild to moderate dementia. (*Exelon, Razadyne*)

Assisted living facility: A *long-term care facility* with on-call nursing staff for individuals who are independent but need help with some activities of daily living.

Ataxia (uh-tak-see-uh): Unsteadiness caused by the brain's failure to regulate the posture as well as the strength and direction of limb movements.

Atrophy (at-rah-fee): A decrease in size or wasting away of a body part or tissue.

Attention deficit: Difficulty maintaining attention, which results in impulsive behavior and excessive activity.

Autonomic nervous system (ANS): The part of the nervous system that regulates key functions of the body, including the activity of the heart muscle, the gastrointestinal tract, the urinary tract, and the glands. The ANS is divided into several systems, including the **inhibitory** and **excitatory systems**. LBD can cause ANS dysfunctions that increase inhibitory effects and decrease excitatory effects, thus causing a slowing down of involuntary functions.

Black box warning: A warning on a medication that is considered so serious that it is surrounded by a black box.

Bradykinesia (brad-e-ki-ZEE-UH): Slowness of movement.

Bradyphrasia (brady-e-FRAY-zh-uh): Slowness of thought.

Brain stem: The stemlike part of the brain that is connected to the spinal cord. The brain stem manages messages going between the brain and the rest of the body, and it controls basic body functions such as breathing, swallowing, heart rate, and blood pressure. The brain stem also controls consciousness and determines whether one is alert or sleepy. The *substantia nigra* is located in this area.

Capgras syndrome: A *delusional misidentification* in which the patient believes that someone close to him (spouse, caregiver) has been replaced by a similar-appearing imposter.

Carbidopa (car-bee-DO-pah): A generic drug used together with *levodopa* to treat the symptoms *Parkinson's disease*. Used alone, it has no effect on Parkinson's symptoms. *(Sinemet)*

Caregiver: An individual who cares for others who have health problems or disabilities.

Catheter: A hollow flexible tube inserted into a body cavity, duct, or vessel to allow the passage of fluids or distend a passageway.

Celebrex: The trade name for **celecoxib** (sel-AH-cok-sib), an anti-inflammatory drug thought to reduce dementia risk in persons with a family history of dementia.

Celexa (sah-LEK-sah): The trade name for **citalopram hydrobromide** (si-tal-oh-pram hī-drō-**brō** mīd), a *selective serotonin reuptake inhibitor (SSRI)* antidepressant medication. *(Desyrel, Paxil, Prozac, selective serotonin reuptake inhibitors, Zoloft)*

Central nervous system (CNS): The part of the nervous system consisting of the brain and spinal cord.

Cerebral: Pertaining to the brain, the cerebrum, or the intellect.

Cerebral cortex: The part of the brain responsible for the processes of thought, perception, and memory and serving as the seat of advanced motor function, social abilities, language, and problem solving.

Cerebrospinal fluid: A watery fluid, continuously produced and absorbed, that flows in the cavities within the brain and around the surface of the brain and spinal cord.

Cerebrovascular disease: A disease of the cerebrum and the blood vessels supplying it; commonly called stroke. Symptoms include *dementia*.

Cerebrovascular system: The system of blood vessels and arteries that supply the brain.

Chloral hydrate (Klor-ul hi-dr-ate): A medication used as a sleeping aid for insomnia.

Clinical trials: Trials to evaluate the effectiveness and safety of medications or medical devices by monitoring their effects on large groups of people.

Cognition: The process of being aware, knowing, thinking, learning, and judging.

Cognitive abilities: The skills used to facilitate memory, executive functions, perception, impulse control, and communication.

Cognitive fluctuations: Fluctuations of arousal and/or cognition, with some hours or days appearing normal or near normal and other periods involving much more severe sleepiness, confusion, disorientation, forgetfulness, and so forth.

Computerized axial tomography (CAT): A type of scan that adds x-ray images with the aid of a computer to generate cross-sectional views of an internal organ or bodily tissues. In dementia cases, CAT scans of the brain are sometimes used to support the diagnosis.

Confabulation: The supplying of ready answers to questions without regard for truth. Patients often fill in gaps in memory with plausible facts.

Convalescent home: See *nursing home*.

Cortex: The outer layer of the cerebrum and cerebellum, which are parts of the brain.

Corticospinal (Kort-tih-ko-SPI-nel): Refers to tissues and fluids that are part of or related to the cerebral cortex and the spinal cord.

Dark joke: A type of humor that makes light of serious and often taboo subjects such as mental illness, with a focus is on the absurd rather than the pitiable. Caregivers often use dark jokes as a coping mechanism to relieve stress.

Deep brain stimulation (DBS): A surgical procedure that is effective in treating Parkinson's disease. The surgery includes the implantation of permanent electrodes in various parts of the brain through which continuous pulses of electricity are given to control the symptoms of Parkinson's disease.

Deficits: The physical and/or cognitive skills or abilities that a person has lost, has difficulty with, or can no longer perform because of his or her dementia.

Delusion: A gross misrepresentation of reality. Typical delusions include those of persecution, romance, grandeur, and control.

Delusional misidentification: The delusional belief that real people or one's own home are replaced by impostors, or that the mirror image of one's self is another person. *(Capgras syndrome)*

Dementia: The impairment of two or more *cognitive abilities*. *Alzheimer's disease* is the most common cause of dementia; LBD and *vascular dementia* are the next most common. Other causes are brain injury, brain tumors, toxicity, encephalitis, meningitis, *fronto-temporal dementia*, syphilis, and thyroid disease.

Dementia with Lewy bodies (DLB): A *Lewy body dementia* in which the cognitive dysfunctions precede motor dysfunctions. Symptoms include cognitive, perceptual, sleep, and autonomic dysfunctions. Closely related to *Parkinson's disease with dementia (PDD)*. It may also be called diffuse Lewy body disease, cortical Lewy body disease, dementia with Lewy body, or Lewy body variant of Alzheimer's disease.

Dementia capable: Describes medical specialists who are skilled in working with people with dementia and their caregivers. They are knowledgeable about the kinds of services that may help caregivers and patients with dementia as well as about which agencies and individuals provide such services.

Depression: An illness involving the body, mood, and thoughts. Symptoms include a loss of interest in life activities, low self-esteem, feelings of helplessness and hopelessness, poor appetite, and weight loss. See also *major depression* and *situational depression*.

Desyrel (Des-ur-ul): The trade name for **trazodone hydrochloride** (traz-uh-doan hi-dro-klor-ide), a non-*SSRI antidepressant* that allows more serotonin to stimulate the nerves in the brain.

Disinhibition: A lack of tact and impulse control.

Dizziness: A painless head discomfort with many possible causes. It is also called lightheadedness, unsteadiness, and vertigo.

Dopamine: An amino acid that occurs as a neurotransmitter in the brain.

Dry mouth: The condition of not having enough saliva to keep the mouth wet, caused by inadequately functioning salivary glands.

Durable power of attorney: A type of advance medical directive in which legal documents provide the power of attorney to another person in the case of an incapacitating medical condition.

Dyskinesia (dis-ki-NEE-zhuh): A condition causing abnormal muscle movement, which can occur as a side effect of certain medications, such as levodopa and antipsychotic drugs.

Dysphagia (dis-fay-suh): Difficulty in swallowing.

Dysphasia (dis-fey-zhuh): A speech impairment caused by lesions in the brain. More severe forms of dysphasia are called aphasia.

Dysphoria (dis-for-ee-ah): A general feeling of anxiety.

Dyspnea (disp-nee-ah): Difficult or labored breathing, or shortness of breath.

Dyspraxia (dis-prak-ee-ah): The impaired or painful function of any organ of the body.

Dystonia (dis-TOE-nee-ah): Involuntary movements and prolonged muscle contraction resulting in twisting body motions, tremor, and abnormal posture. These movements may involve the entire body or only an isolated area.

Elder law attorney: An attorney who practices in the area of elder law, which focuses on issues typically affecting older adults.

End stage: The last phase in the course of a progressive disease.

Euphoria (you-FOR-ee-uh): A persistent and unreasonable sense of well-being.

Excessive daytime somnolence (EDS): The tendency to fall asleep intermittently during the day. It is also called excessive daytime sleepiness.

Executive functions: The skills used for reasoning, problem solving, judgment, learning, and sequential tasks.

Exelon: The trade name for **rivastigmine** (ri-veh-STIG-meen), an acetylcholinesterase inhibitor. The Exelon skin patch bypasses the gastrointestinal tract to reduce gastrointestinal (GI) side effects.

Facial affect: The expression that shows on one's face. *(mask-like face)*

Familial: An attribute that tends to occur more frequently in family members than is possible by chance. A familial disease may be genetic or environmental.

Family or general physician: A medical doctor who provides continuing and comprehensive health care for the individual and family. This is usually the first physician a patient sees before being referred to a specific specialist.

Festination: Walking in rapid, short, and shuffling steps.

Florinef (Flor-i-nef): The trade name for **fludrocortisone acetate** (flu·dro·cor·ti·sone as-i-teyt), a medication used to treat orthostatic hypotension.

Flushing: An involuntary response of the nervous system leading to a temporary widening of the capillaries of the involved skin. It is usually caused by excitement, exercise, fever, or embarrassment, but can also be caused by medications that widen the capillaries, such as niacin.

Foley catheter: A flexible plastic tube (catheter) inserted into the bladder to provide drainage of urine on a continuous basis.

Fronto-temporal dementia: A form of dementia caused by a shrinkage of the frontal and temporal lobes of the brain. It is also called **Pick's disease**. Sometimes *hereditary*, it is characterized by a slowly progressive deterioration of social skills and changes in personality leading to impairment of intellect, memory, and language. This type of dementia results in behavior problems, including severe apathy and lack of compassion or empathy.

Gait: The manner of walking. People with dementia often have reduced gait, meaning their ability to lift their feet as they walk has diminished.

Generic drug: A drug that is produced and distributed without patent protection. Generic drugs are usually much less expensive than brand-name drugs.

Geriatric: Pertaining to the elderly.

Gerontology: The study of the aging process, including physical, mental, and social changes. A **gerontologist** is a person with a master's degree or doctorate in gerontology.

Glutamate: A neurotransmitter that facilitates cognitive and perceptive functions.

Guardian: An individual appointed by the courts who is authorized to make legal and financial decisions for another individual.

Haldol (hal-dol): The trade name for **haloperidol** (Hal-oh-PER-dol), *antipsychotic drug*. It is particularly dangerous for LBD patients.

Hallucination: A sensory experience in which a person can perceive what is not there. Visual hallucinations are the most common with LBD. Hallucinations can also be auditory (hearing), gustatory (taste), kinesthetic (body movement), Lilliputian (people and things appearing smaller than normal), musical (auditory hallucination concerning music), olfactory (smell), or tactile (touch).

Heredity, hereditary: The genetic transmission of characteristics from parent to child.

Home health care: The provision of skilled heath care and custodial health aides services in the home on a part-time basis for the treatment of an illness or injury. Home health care is covered under Medicare Part A and Medicare Part B, provided it is prescribed by a physician. Durable medical equipment is also covered when provided by a home health agency. A **home health agency** provides services such as skilled nursing care, physical therapy, occupational therapy, speech therapy, and care by home health aides.

Hospice: A program or facility that provides *palliative care* for people who are near the end of life and for their families. Hospice care can be provided at home, in a hospice or another freestanding facility, or within a hospital. Hospice care is designed to provide care to people in the final phase of a terminal illness and is focused on comfort and quality of life rather than cure. The philosophy of hospice is to provide support for the patient's emotional, social, and spiritual needs as well as medical symptoms as part of treating the whole person.

Hypokinesia (hi-poh-ki-NEE-zhuh): An abnormal decrease in muscular movement.

Idiopathic: A condition that starts without apparent cause.

Illusions: The perception that objects appear different from what they actually are.

Incontinence: The inability to control excretions. Urinary incontinence is the inability to keep urine in the bladder, and fecal incontinence is the inability to retain feces in the rectum.

Insomnia: The chronic perception or complaint of inadequate or poor-quality sleep because of one or more of the following: difficulty falling asleep, waking up frequently during the night with difficulty returning to sleep, waking up too early in the morning, or unrefreshing sleep.

Instrumental activities of daily living (IADL): The secondary level of activities during daily living, such as cooking, writing, and driving.

Intention tremor: A tremor occurring when a person attempts voluntary movement.

Irritability: The state of being easily annoyed, causing testiness.

Klonopin (klon-uh-pin): The trade name for **clonazepam** (klo-NAZ-uh-pam), an antianxiety drug used to treat REM sleep behavior disorder.

Levodopa: A generic drug used, together with *carbidopa*, to treat the symptoms of *Parkinson's disease*. Used alone, it causes adverse side effects. *(Sinemet)*

Lewy bodies: Small round clumps of normal proteins that for unknown reasons become abnormally clumped together inside neurons.

Lewy body dementia (LBD): Dementia caused by Lewy bodies in the brain. It includes both *dementia with Lewy bodies (DLB)* and *Parkinson's disease with dementia (PDD)*, and is closely related to *Parkinson's disease* and *multiple system atrophy (MSA)*.

Living will: A legal document in which the signer requests not to be kept alive by medical life support or life-prolonging systems in the event of a terminal illness.

Long-term care (LTC): Personal care services given at home or in a *skilled nursing facility* for people with chronic disabilities and lengthy illnesses. Medicare does not generally cover long-term care.

Long-term care facility (LTCF): A facility that provides rehabilitative, restorative, and/or ongoing skilled nursing care to patients or residents in need of assistance with activities of daily living.

Long-term care ombudsman: An advocate who resolves disputes between residents of skilled nursing facilities or assisted living care facilities and the facility management. This individual also works to inform residents and their family members of their rights and protections while residing in a facility.

Magnetic resonance imaging (MRI): A radiology technique designed to image internal structures of the body using magnetism, radio waves, and a computer to produce the images of body structures. The image and resolution are detailed and can detect tiny changes of structures within the body, particularly in the soft tissue, brain and spinal cord, abdomen, and joints.

Major depression: A disease that interferes with the ability to work, sleep, eat, and enjoy once pleasurable activities. It often includes suicidal thoughts.

Masklike face: A condition in which *facial affect* shows little or no sense of animation. It is seen in *Parkinson's disease.*

Medicaid: State programs of public assistance to persons regardless of age whose income and resources are insufficient to pay for health care. The U.S. federal government provides matching funds to state Medicaid programs.

Medicare: The U.S. government's health insurance program for individuals 65 years of age or older, and certain younger people with specific disabilities or end-stage renal disease. Part A covers inpatient hospital stays, Part B covers physician and outpatient services, and Part D covers prescription drugs.

Melatonin: An herbal supplement used to treat sleep disorders such as insomnia.

Memory: The ability to or process of storing, encoding, and retrieving information. **Short-term** (or working) **memory** temporarily stores and manages information required to carry out complex cognitive tasks such as learning, reasoning, and comprehension. **Long-term memory** permanently stores, manages, and retrieves information for later use. Items of information stored as long-term memory may be available for a lifetime.

Memory span: The number of items, usually words or numbers, that a person can retain and recall. Memory span is a test of short-term memory function. The average item span for normal adults is seven.

Mini-Mental State Examination (MMSE): An examination for determining the mental status of a person. Performed by a health care professional, the test measures a person's basic cognitive skills, such as short-term memory, long-term memory, orientation, writing, and language.

Mirapex (MIR-uh-peks)**:** The trade name for **pramipexole** (pram-uh-pek-sole), a medication used to treat Parkinson's disease. It helps replace the neurotransmitter dopamine.

Multiple system atrophy (MSA): A rare, always terminal, degenerative neurological disorder characterized by a combination of parkinsonism, cerebellar or corticospinal signs, pyramidal signs, and dysautonomia.

Namenda (nah-MEN-dah): The trade name for **memantine hydrochloride** (meh-man-teen hi-dro-klor-ide), a dementia drug that works with the neurotransmitter *glutamate*. Although seldom used alone with LBD, it is useful as an adjunct to *acetylcholinesterase inhibitors*.

National Institutes of Health (NIH): A US health agency devoted to medical research. It consists of more than 20 separate institutes and centers, including *NINDS*, and *NIA*.

National Institute of Neurological Disorders and Stroke (NINDS): A NIH agency with the mission of researching nervous system disorders for causes, prevention, diagnosis, and treatment.

National Institute on Aging (NIA): A *NIH* agency with the mission of researching the biomedical, social, and behavioral aspects of the aging processes to promote prevention of age-related diseases and disabilities and a better quality of life for the elderly.

Nerve: A bundle of fibers that uses chemical and electrical signals to transmit sensory and motor information from one body part to another.

Neurodegenerative: Causing degeneration of nervous tissue.

Neuroleptic drug: See *antipsychotic drugs*.

Neuroleptic sensitivity: A reaction to a *neuroleptic drug* causing side effects including increased confusion, rigidity, immobility, and an inability to perform tasks or to communicate. The reaction may or may not be permanent. The sensitivity is present in at least 50% of LBD patients; with use of traditional antipsychotic drugs increasing morbidity twofold to threefold.

Neurological: Related to the nerves or the nervous system, including the brain, spinal cord, and nerves.

Neurology: A medical specialty concerned with the diagnosis and treatment of disorders of the nervous system. A **neurologist** is a physician who specializes in the diagnosis and treatment of disorders of the nervous system. A **neuropsychiatrist** is a *psychiatrist* who specializes in neurology. A **neuropsychologist** is a psychologist who has completed special training in neurology and who diagnoses and treats neurological illnesses using a predominantly medical approach.

Neuron: Nerve cell that sends and receives electrical signals over long distances within the body.

Neurontin: The trade name for **gabapentin** (gab-ah-PEN-tin), an anticonvulsive drug used to treat *restless legs syndrome.*

Neuropathy: Any and all diseases or malfunctions of the nerves. A **neuropathologist** is a *pathologist* who specializes in the diagnosis of diseases of the brain and nervous system by microscopic examination of the tissue and other means.

Neuropsychological testing: The assessment of cognitive abilities such as memory, attention, orientation to time and place, use of language, ability to carry out various tasks, and ability to follow instructions.

Neurotransmitter: A chemical released from a nerve cell that transmits an impulse from one nerve cell to another nerve cell, muscle, organ, or other tissue. A neurotransmitter is a messenger of neurological information from one cell to another.

Nightmares: A dream that arouses feelings of intense fear, horror, or distress.

Nurse: A person trained, licensed, or skilled in nursing.

Nurse, licensed practical (LPN) or licensed vocational (LVN): A nurse who has completed a 1- or 2-year training program in health care and earned a state license. LPNs provide direct patient care for people with chronic illness in nursing homes, hospitals, and home settings. They assist RNs in caring for acutely ill patients.

Nurse, registered (RN): A nurse who has completed a 2- to 4-year degree program in nursing and provides direct patient care for acutely or chronically ill patients. RNs may further specialize in a particular area.

Nurse practitioner (NP): A registered nurse (RN) who has completed an advanced training program in a medical specialty such as pediatrics or internal medicine. This individual may function as a primary direct provider of health care and can prescribe medications.

Nursing assistant (NA): A person who has completed a brief health care training program and who provides support services for RNs and LPNs. Also known as an orderly or, when certified by a state agency, a certified nurse aide (CNA).

Nursing home: A residential facility for persons with chronic illness or disability, particularly older people who have mobility and eating problems. Also called a *convalescent home, long-term care facility,* or a *skilled nursing facility.*

Occupational therapist (OT): A professional who works with anyone who has a permanent or temporary impairment in physical or mental functioning. The aim of occupational therapy is to help clients perform daily tasks in their living and working environments and assist them in developing the skills to live independent, satisfying, and productive lives.

Orthostatic hypotension: Temporary lowering of blood pressure (hypotension) usually caused by suddenly standing up (orthostatic). The change in position causes a temporary reduction in blood flow and therefore a shortage of oxygen to the brain. This leads to lightheadedness and, sometimes, *syncope*.

Palliative care: Care that relieves pain but does not cure or change the path of the disease. Palliative services are among those offered by *hospice*.

Paranoia: Suspiciousness or mistrust exhibited by patients with dementia as their memory becomes worse. For example, a patient misplaces a possession but believes it has been stolen.

Parasympathetic nervous system (PNS): A part of the autonomic nervous system that slows the heart rate, increases intestinal and gland activity, and relaxes sphincter muscles.

Parkinson's disease (PD): A slowly progressive neurologic disease characterized by a fixed, inexpressive face; tremor at rest; slowing of voluntary movements; a gait with short accelerating steps; peculiar posture; and muscle weakness. PD is caused by degeneration of an area of the brain called the basal ganglia and low production of the neurotransmitter dopamine.

Parkinson's disease with dementia (PDD): A dementia that appears after a person has had Parkinson's disease for at least a year. The cause and symptoms are those of *dementia with Lewy bodies* and *Parkinson's disease* together.

Parkinsonian symptoms: Movement dysfunctions in an individual who may not be diagnosed with *Parkinson's disease*.

Parkinsonism: Movement dysfunctions caused by drugs used to treat other conditions.

Pathologist: A physician who specializes in the diagnosis of disease by microscopic examination of the tissue and other means.

Paxil (pak-sil): The trade name for **paroxetine** (pa-rok-si-teen), a SSRI *antidepressant*. *(Celexa, Desyrel, Prozac, selective serotonin reuptake inhibitors, Zoloft)*

Perception: The mind's interpretation of sensory input from vision, hearing, smell, touch and taste.

Physical therapist (PT): A person trained and certified by a state or accrediting body to design and implement physical therapy programs. Physical therapists may work within a hospital or clinic; in a school, providing assistance to special education students; or as an independent practitioner.

Physical therapy (PT): A branch of rehabilitative health that uses specially designed exercises and equipment to help patients regain or improve their physical abilities.

Physician: A person trained in the art of healing. Physicians are also referred to as a medical doctor or MD.

Physician assistant (PA): A mid-level medical practitioner who works under the supervision of a licensed doctor (an MD) or osteopathic physician (a DO).

Plaques: Lesions of brain tissue found along with *tangles* in Alzheimer's disease.

Positron emission tomography (PET): A highly specialized imaging technique that uses short-lived radioactive substances to produce three-dimensional colored images (PET scans) of metabolic activity or body functions. The PET scan has been used to assess adult dementia.

Postural instability: The inability to maintain a correct posture in either a standing or sitting position.

ProAmatine (pro-AM-uh-teen): The trade name for **midodrine hydrochloride** (mi-deh-dreen hi-dro-klor-ide), a medication that can be used to treat *orthostatic hypotension.*

Progressive: Increasing in scope or severity.

Progressive supranuclear palsy (PSP): A neurological disorder of unknown origin that gradually destroys cells in many areas of the brain, leading to serious and permanent problems with the control of gait and balance. Patients also often show alterations of mood and behavior, including depression and apathy as well as progressive mild dementia.

Propulsive gait: A disturbance of *gait* that causes steps to become faster and faster with progressively shorter steps that pass from a walking to a running pace and may precipitate falling forward.

Protein: A large molecule composed of one or more chains of amino acids in a specific order determined by the base sequence of nucleotides in the DNA coding for the protein. Proteins are required for the structure, function, and regulation of the body's cells, tissues, and organs. Each protein has unique functions. Proteins are essential components of muscles, skin, bones, and the body as a whole.

Provigil: The trade name for **modafinil** (mō-dăf-ĭ-nĭl), a *psychostimulant drug* used to treat excessive daytime sleepiness or problems with breathing while asleep. It may also improve alertness in dementia patients and is considered less addictive than other psychostimulants.

Prozac (pro-zak): The trade name for **fluoxetine hydrochloride** (flew-ox-eh-teen hi-dro-klor-ide), a SSRI *antidepressant. (Celexa, Desyrel, Paxil, selective serotonin reuptake inhibitors, Zoloft)*

Psychiatry: A medical specialty concerned with the prevention, diagnosis, and treatment of mental illness. A **psychiatrist** is a physician who specializes in psychiatry.

Psychiatric illness: Mental illness. A psychological or behavioral pattern associated with distress or disability that occurs in an individual and is not a part of normal development or culture.

Psychology: The study of the mind and mental processes, especially in relation to behavior. A **psychologist** is a person with a master's or doctorate in psychology who uses talk or behavioral therapy as treatment. Psychologists cannot prescribe medication but usually work closely with a physician or psychiatrist who can. **Psychological** refers to mind and mental processes.

Psychomotor: Of or relating to movement or muscular activity associated with mental processes.

Psychopharmacology: The management of psychiatric illness using medication such as antidepressants, antipsychotics, and antianxiety drugs.

Psychosis: A mental illness that markedly interferes with a person's capacity to meet life's everyday demands. Symptoms can include seeing, hearing, smelling, or tasting things that are not there, paranoia, and delusional thoughts.

Psychotic: Pertaining to psychosis as in "psychotic behavior."

Psychostimulant drug: A medication used to increase psychomotor activity. It can improve concentration and impulse control in attention deficit hyperactivity disorder. Many are addictive. *(Provigil)*

Rapid eye movement (REM) sleep: The portion of sleep when the eyes move rapidly, causing the lids to flutter. Dreams occur during REM sleep. *(REM sleep behavior disorder)*

Razadyne (raz-eh-dine): The trade name for **galantamine hydrobromide** (gah-lan-teh-men hī-drō-**brō** mīd) and formerly known as **Reminyl**. It is an *acetylcholinesterase inhibitor* that is used to treat mild or moderate dementia. *(Aricept, Exelon)*

Receptor: A structure on the surface of a nerve cell (or inside a cell) that receives and responds to stimuli.

REM sleep behavior disorder (RBD): A sleep disorder in which sleep paralysis, which normally disables the voluntary muscles during *rapid eye movement (REM) sleep*, fails to occur, resulting in the dreamer acting out movements, especially during dramatic episodes, with possible injurious results to bed partner.

Respite program: Time that enables a person to take needed breaks from being a caregiver.

Restless leg syndrome (RLS): An uncontrollable urge to move legs to relieve uncomfortable sensations such as creeping, tingling, twitching, throbbing, or prickling. The sensations typically become more noticeable with rest (sitting or lying down) and ease with motion. *(Neurontin, Tegretol)*

Retropulsion: The tendency to fall or move backwards.

Rigidity: Increased muscle tone in neck, arms, or legs, causing stiffness or inability to move.

Risperdal (ris-per-dal): The trade name for **risperidone** (rĭ-**spâr**-ə-dōn'), an *atypical antipsychotic* medication. *(antipsychotic drugs, Seroquel)*

Sedative drug: Medication that acts to assist sleep by depressing the central nervous system. It may cause serious side effects for LBD patients and is often very addictive. *(Ambien, Lunesta)*

Selective serotonin reuptake inhibitor (SSRI): *Antidepressant drug* used to treat depression, panic attacks, and other anxiety disorders. They restore the balance of *neurotransmitters* in the brain, thereby improving mood and feeling of well-being, without depleting *acetylcholine*. These drugs are the drug of choice for patients with LBD. *(Celexa, Paxil, Prozac, Zoloft)*

Seroquel (ser-ō-kwĕl): The trade name for **quetiapine** (kwət-ī-ə-pēn), an *atypical antipsychotic*. Insomnia can also be treated with this drug. This is often the antipsychotic of choice for LBD patients. *(Risperdal)*

Serotonin: A *neurotransmitter* found in the brain and known to influence mood.

Sinemet (sin-eh-met): The trade name for a combination of *carbidopa* and *levodopa*, which is used to control motor dysfunctions.

Single photon emission computed tomography (SPECT scan): A nuclear medicine procedure in which a gamma camera rotates around the patient and takes pictures from many angles, which a computer then uses to form a tomographic (cross-sectional) image.

Situational depression: Temporary symptoms of depression that occur as a reaction to stressful life events. The symptoms tend to leave when life becomes less stressful.

Skilled nursing facility (SNF): An institution providing persons older than 65 years of age (and younger disabled persons) with daily skilled nursing care, rehabilitation, and other medical services.

Sleep apnea: The temporary halting of breathing during sleep, often resulting in daytime sleepiness.

Somnolent: Sleepy or sleep inducing. *(excessive daytime somnolence)*

Spatial disorientation: Difficulty navigating in familiar surroundings.

Stages: The course of a disease progression defined by levels or periods of severity: early, mild, moderate, moderately severe, and severe.

Substantia nigra: A layer of large, pigmented nerve cells in the mid-brain that produces dopamine and whose destruction is associated with Parkinson's disease. *(dopamine, Parkinson's disease)*

Sympathetic nervous system: A part of the autonomic nervous system that accelerates the heart rate, constricts blood vessels, and raises blood pressure.

Synapse: A point of connection (or communication) between two nerve cells.

Syncope: The partial or complete loss of consciousness. Recovery is spontaneous.

Tangles: Twisted fibers that build up around nerve cells of patients with *Alzheimer's disease. (plaques)*

Tegretol (teg-ruh-tol)**:** The trade name for **carbamazepine** (kar-bah-ma-zuh-pen), an anticonvulsive drug sometimes used to treat mental illness, *depression*, and *restless legs syndrome. (Neurontin)*

Tremor: Any abnormal repetitive shaking, often involving the fingers, arms, or legs. An **active, essential,** or **intentional tremor** occurs when movement is initiated, such as when writing or lifting a cup. It is the most common type of tremor and also the most commonly observed movement disorder. A **passive** or **resting tremor** occurs when the body is at rest and diminishes or stops during voluntary movement.

Vascular dementia: A common form of *dementia* caused by *cerebrovascular disease*, which resulted from a series of small strokes, each of which causes a small loss of cognitive functions. Symptoms include confusion, memory loss, *incontinence*, loss of *executive functions*, and inappropriate displays of emotion. Vascular dementia commonly begins between the ages of 60 and 75 and affects men more often than women.

Verbal blocking: Difficulty in expressing full sentences and losing track of one's thoughts.

Visuospatial function: A cognitive function related to the combination of visual and spatial awareness. It is also called hand–eye coordination.

Zoloft (zō-lôft')**:** The trade name for **sertraline** (sər-trə-lēn), a *selective serotonin reuptake inhibitor (SSRI) antidepressant* used to treat depression, panic attacks, and other anxiety-type disorders. *(Celexa, Desyrel, Paxil, Prozac, selective serotonin reuptake inhibitors)*

Zyprexa (zi-prex-see-uh)**:** The trade name for **olanzapine** (ə-lăn-zə-pēn')*,* an *atypical antipsychotic* that has not been shown to be safe or effective treatment for elderly people with dementia. *(Seroquel, Risperdal)*

Acronyms

Although many of these acronyms do not appear in the text of this book, you may come across them as you read other materials and talk to professionals.

AAN	American Academy of Neurology
ACh-E	acetylcholine esterase
AChEIs	acetylcholinesterase inhibitors
ACh-R	acetylcholine receptor
AD	Alzheimer disease
ADAS-Cog	Alzheimer's Disease Assessment Scale-Cognitive subscale
ADC	Alzheimer's Disease Center
ADEAR	Alzheimer's Disease Education and Referral Center
ADL	activities of daily living (also see IADL)
ADRC	Alzheimer's Disease Research Center
ADRDA	Alzheimer's Disease and Related Disorders Association
ALF	assisted living facility
ANS	autonomic nervous system (also see S-ANS and P-ANS)
AS	α-synuclein (alpha-synuclein)
BNT	Boston Naming Test
BS	bachelor of science degree
CAMCOG	Cambridge Cognitive Examination
CAMDEX	Cambridge Examination for Mental Disorders of the Elderly
CANTAB	Cambridge Neuropsychological Test Automated Battery

CAT	computerized axial tomography
CBD	corticobasal degeneration
CDC	Centers for Disease Control and Prevention
CDR	Clinical Dementia Rating [scale]
CG	caregiver
ChAT	cortical choline acetyltransferase
ChE-I	cholinesterase inhibitor
CJD	Creutzfeldt-Jakob disease
CLBD	cortical Lewy body disease (see LBD)
CMS	Center for Medicare & Medicaid Services (U.S. government agency)
CNA	certified nursing assistant
CNS	central nervous system
COMT	catechol-O-methyltransferase
CPR	cardiopulmonary resuscitation
CSH	carotid sinus hypersensitivity
CSS	carotid sinus syndrome
CT	computed tomography [scan]
CVD	cerebrovascular disease
CVLT	California Verbal Learning Test
DAT	dopamine transporter
DBS	deep brain stimulation
DLB	dementia with Lewy bodies (see LBD)
DLBD	diffuse Lewy body disease (see LBD)
DNR	do not resuscitate
DRS	Dementia Rating Scale
DSM	*Diagnostic and Statistical Manual of Mental Disorders*
DSM-IV	*Diagnostic and Statistical Manual of Mental Disorders, Fourth Edition*
ECG	electrocardiogram
ECT	electroconvulsive therapy
EEG	electroencephalogram
EKG	elektrokardiogramm (German)
EPS	extrapyramidal motor symptoms
EOG	electrooculogram
ET	essential tremor
FDA	Food and Drug Administration
FRCP	Fellow of the Royal College of Physicians

FTD	frontotemporal dementia
FTDP-17	frontotemporal dementia with parkinsonism related to chromosome 17
HD	Huntington disease
HVLT	Hopkins Verbal Learning Test
IADL	instrumental activities of daily living
IBS	irritable bowel syndrome
ICD	*International Classification of Diseases* (World Health Organization)
ICD-9	*International Classification of Diseases, Ninth Revision* (Symptom Checklist for Mental Disorders)
IHC	immunohistochemistry
IU	international unit of drug
IV	(*a*) intravenous; (*b*) roman numeral 4 as in 4th edition
LB	Lewy bodies
LBD	Lewy body dementia, also known as Lewy body disease, dementia with Lewy bodies, diffuse Lewy body disease, cortical Lewy body disease
LBDA	Lewy Body Dementia Association, Inc.
LBV	Lewy body variant
LCPC	licensed clinical professional counselor
LN	Lewy neuritis
LPN	licensed practical nurse
LTC	long-term care
LTCF	long-term care facility
LTHC	long-term health care
LVN	licensed vocational nurse
MAOI	monoamine oxidase inhibitor
MCI	mild cognitive impairment
MD	doctor of medicine
MG	myasthenia gravis
MIBG	iodine-131-meta-iodobenzylguanidine
MID	multi-infarct dementia
MMSE	Mini-Mental State Examination
MPH	master of public health [degree]
MRI	magnetic resonance imaging
MRS	magnetic resonance spectroscopy
MSA	multiple system atrophy
MS	multiple sclerosis

MS	master of science (degree [also MSc])
nAChR	nicotinic acetylcholine receptors
NCVI	neurocardiovascular instability
NFT	neurofibrillary tangles
NIA	National Institute on Aging
NIA-RI	National Institute on Aging and Reagan Institute
NIH	National Institutes of Health
NIMH	National Institute of Mental Health
NINCDS	National Institute of Neurological and Communicative Disorders and Stroke
NINDS	National Institute of Neurological Disorders and Stroke
NMS	neuroleptic malignant syndrome
NP	nurse practitioner
NPF	National Parkinson Foundation
NPI	Neuro-Psychiatric Inventory
OH	orthostatic hypotension
OSA	obstructive sleep apnea
OT	occupational therapist
OTC	over-the-counter
PA	physician assistant
PAF	pure autonomic failure
P-ANS	parasympathetic autonomic nervous system
PD	Parkinson disease
PDD	Parkinson disease with dementia
PDF	Parkinson's Disease Foundation
PET	positron emission tomography [scan]
PhD	doctoral research degree
PIGD	postural instability and gait disorder (or difficulty)
PKAN	pantothenate kinase-associated neurodegeneration
PLM	periodic limb movement
PPI	prepulse inhibition
PSMS	Physical Self-Maintenance Scale
PSP	progressive supranuclear palsy
PT	physical therapy
RBD	rapid eye movement (REM) sleep behavior disorder
REM	rapid eye movement
RLS	restless legs syndrome
RN	registered nurse

RT	resting tremor
S-ANS	sympathetic autonomic nervous system
SDLT	senile dementia of Lewy body type (see LBD)
SIVD	subcortical ischemic vascular dementia
SNCA	α-synuclein (alpha-synuclein) gene
SNF	skilled nursing facility
SPECT	single photon emission computed tomography
SSRI	selective serotonin reuptake inhibitor
TD	tardive dyskinesia
TIA	transient ischemic attack
UPDRS	Unified Parkinson's Disease Rating Scale
VA	Veterans Affairs
VaD	vascular dementia
VCD	vascular cognitive disorder
VCI	vascular cognitive impairment
VCI-ND	vascular cognitive impairment no dementia
VCJD	variant Creutzfeldt-Jakob disease
VH	visual hallucinations

Online Resources

Associations

Alzheimer's Association: http://www.alz.org/

Alzheimer's Foundation of America: http://www.alzfdn.org

Alzheimer's Disease Education & Referral (ADEAR) Center: http://www.alzheimers.org

American Parkinson Disease Association: http://www.apdaparkinson.org

Lewy Body Dementia Association: http://www.lbda.org/

Michael J. Fox Foundation for Parkinson's Research: http://michaeljfox.org

National Parkinson Foundation: http://www.parkinson.org

Parkinson's Disease Foundation: http://www.pdf.org

Caregiver Services

Assist Guide Information Services: http://www.agis.com/

The Beatitudes Campus: http://beatitudescampus.org

ElderCare Online: http://www.cc-online.net/

Family Caregiver Alliance: http://www.caregiver.org

Full Circle of Care: http://www.fullcirclecare.org

Helpguide, Preventing Caregiver Burnout: http://helpguide.org/elder /caring _for_caregivers.htm

National Association of Area Agencies on Aging: http://www.n4a.org/

National Family Caregivers Association: http://www.nfcacares.org

Medicare: http://www.medicare.gov

Medication Research

DoubleCheckMD: http://www.doublecheckmd.com/

Healthline: Drug Interaction Checker: http://www.healthline.com
/druginteractions

Lewy Body Dementia Association Clinical Trials Information:
http://www.lbda.org/category/3514/clinical-trials.htm

MedlinePlus: http://www.nlm.nih.gov/medlineplus/druginformation.html

WebMD: http://www.webmd.com/drugs/index-drugs.aspx

Forums

Lewy Body Dementia Association forums: http://community.lbda.org/forum/

Yahoo Lewy body dementia Groups:

http://www.groups.yahoo.com/group/LBDcaregivers/join

http://www.groups.yahoo.com/group/LBD_caringspouses/join

References

Chapter 1

1. Ferman TJ. Dementia with Lewy bodies: a review of clinical diagnosis, neuropathology and management options. *Jacksonville Medical Magazine.* February 2000. Available at: http://www.dcmsonline.org/jax-medicine/2000journals/February2000/lewybodies.htm. Accessed August 23, 2010.

2. Hobson J, Meara J. The detection of dementia and cognitive impairment in a community population of elderly people with Parkinson's disease by use of the CAMCOG neuropsychological test. *Age Ageing.* 1999;28(1): 39–43. Available at: http://ageing.oxfordjournals.org/cgi/reprint/28/1/39.pdf. Accessed August 23, 2010.

Chapter 2

1. Lewy Body Dementia Association, Inc. Virtual groups. Available at: http://www.lbda.org/category/3931/internet-support-groups.htm. Accessed August 23, 2010.

2. LBDA Telephone Helpline, 1-800-LEWYSOS (1-800-539-9767).

Chapter 3

1. The Nutrition Source. Staying active: every body's path to better health. Harvard School of Public Medicine Web site. Available at: http://www.hsph.harvard.edu/nutritionsource/staying-active/staying-active-full-story/index.html. Accessed August 23, 2010.

2. Spencer P. Why people with dementia need daily exercise. *Caring.com.* July 11, 2008. Available at: http://www.caring.com/blogs/caring-currents/exercise-and-dementia. Accessed August 23, 2010.

3. Fernandez A. Combine physical and mental exercise for brain health—interview with Dr. Kramer. *SharpBrains*. 2008. Available at: http://ezinearticles.com/?Combine-Physical-and-Mental-Exercise-For-Brain-Health–Interview-With-Dr-Kramer&id51417007. Accessed August 23, 2010.

4. Fernando A. Build your cognitive reserve—Yaakov Stern. *SharpBrains*. July 23, 2007. Available at: http://www.sharpbrains.com/blog/2007/07/23/build-your-cognitive-reserve-yaakov-stern. Accessed August 23, 2010.

5. Hitti M, Chang L. 3 diet keys to reducing dementia. *WebMD Health News*. November 12, 2007. Available at: http://www.webmd.com/alzheimers/news/20071112/3-diet-keys-to-reducing-dementia. Accessed August 23, 2010.

6. Morgenthaler J. Coenzyme Q10—life giving energy at the cellular level. *SmartPublications*. 2008. Available at: http://www.smart-publications.com/heart_attacks/Coenzyme_Q10.php. Accessed August 23, 2010.

7. Louden K. High-dose vitamin E slows functional decline in Alzheimer's disease. *Medscape Medical News*. May 5, 2009. Available at: http://www.medscape.com/viewarticle/702333. Accessed August 23, 2010.

8. Boyles S, Chang L. Ginkgo biloba doesn't prevent dementia. *WebMD Health News*. November 18, 2008. Available at: http://www.webmd.com/alzheimers/news/20081118/ginkgo-biloba-doesnt-prevent-dementia. Accessed August 23, 2010.

Chapter 4

1. Bechara A. The neurology of social cognition. *Brain*. 2002;125(8):1673–1675. Available at: http://brain.oxfordjournals.org/cgi/content/full/125/8/1673. Accessed August 23, 2010.

2. U.S. Food and Drug Administration. FDA approves generic Aricept to treat dementia related to Alzheimer's disease. Available at: http://www.fda.gov/NewsEvents/Newsroom/PressAnnouncements/ucm194173.htm. Accessed August 23, 2010.

3. Miyasaki JM, Shannon K, Voon V, Ravina B, et al. Practice parameter: evaluation and treatment of depression, psychosis, and dementia in Parkinson disease (an evidence-based review). *Neurology*. 2006;66:996–1002. Available at: http://www.neurology.org/cgi/content/abstract/66/7/996. Accessed August 23, 2010.

4. Tortorice K. Drug class review: cholinesterase inhibitors. U.S. Department of Veteran's Affairs Web site. Available at: http://www.pbm.va.gov/reviews/CholinestInh.pdf. Accessed August 23, 2010.

5. Hitti M, Chang L. FDA OKs 1st Alzheimer's skin patch. *WebMD Health News*. 2007. Available at: http://www.webmd.com/alzheimers/news/20070709 /fda-oks-1st-alzheimers-skin-patch. Accessed August 23, 2010.

6. U.S. Food and Drug Administration. Generic drug roundup: February 2009; Galantamine. *Consumer Health Information*. February 2009. Available at: http://www.fda.gov/consumer/updates/generics020209.html#Galantamine. Accessed August 23, 2010.

7. Richard R. ICPDMD: Drug improves symptoms in two dementias. *MedpageTODAY*. June 12, 2009. Available at: http://www.medpagetoday .com/Neurology/GeneralNeurology/14680. Accessed August 23, 2010.

Chapter 5

1. Haines CD, ed. Parkinson's disease: drug treatments. *WebMD*. June 1, 2005. Available at: http://www.webmd.com/parkinsons-disease/drug-treatments. Accessed August 23, 2010.

Chapter 6

1. Mayo Clinic staff. Restless legs syndrome: treatments and drugs. *Mayo-Clinic.com*. December 23, 2009. Available at: http://www.mayoclinic.com /health/restless-legs-syndrome/DS00191/DSECTION=treatments-and-drugs. Accessed August 23, 2010.

2. Buchfuhrer M. Ask the doctor [Restless Leg Syndrome Foundation Web site]. August 2000. Available at: http://www.rls.org/Document.Doc?&id=798. Accessed August 23, 2010.

3. Hinds L. About the brain. Faculty Page, University of Hawaii, Honolulu Community College Web site. Available at: http://home.honolulu.hawaii .edu/~leilani/brain.html. Accessed August 23, 2010.

Chapter 7

1. Ferman T. Dementia with Lewy bodies: a review of clinical diagnosis, neuropathology and management options. Jacksonville Medicine. 2000. Available at: http://www.dcmsonline.org/jax-medicine/2000journals /February2000/lewybodies.htm. Accessed August 23, 2010.

Chapter 8

1. Memory and Aging Center. Frontotemporal dementia: medications to be avoided. UCSF Memory and Aging Center Web site. November 20, 2008. Available at: http://memory.ucsf.edu/ftd/medical/treatment/avoid/single. Accessed August 23, 2010.

2. Hoyle B. Cholinesterase inhibitors. *Gale Encyclopedia of Neurological Disorders.* 2005. Available at: http://www.encyclopedia.com/doc /1G2-3435200094.html. Accessed August 23, 2010.

3. Memory and Aging Center. Frontotemporal dementia: medications to be avoided. UCSF Memory and Aging Center Web site. November 20, 2008. Available at: http://memory.ucsf.edu/ftd/medical/treatment/avoid/multiple. Accessed August 23, 2010.

4. Doty L Lewy body dementia. AlzOnline. Available at: http://alzonline .phhp.ufl.edu/en/reading/lewybody.php. Accessed August 23, 2010.

5. Boylan LS, Hirsch S. Motor worsening and tardive dyskinesia with aripiprazole in Lewy body dementia. *BMJ Case Reports.* 2009. Abstract. Available at: http://casereports.bmj.com/cgi/content/abstract/2009/jan27_1 /bcr0620080205. Accessed August 23, 2010.

6. Purse M. Antipsychotic medications: black box warning. *About.com Guide.* March 5, 2009. Available at: http://bipolar.about.com/od/antipsychotics/a /1blackbox.htm. Accessed August 23, 2010.

7. Meeks TW, Jeste DV. Beyond the black box: what is the role for antipsychotics in dementia? *Curr Psychiatr.* June 2008;7(6):50–65. Available at: http://www.ncbi.nlm.nih.gov/pmc/articles/PMC2641030/ Accessed August 23, 2010.

8. Lovato J, Williamson J, Atkinson H, et al. Commonly used medications associated with impaired physical function in older adults. *ScienceDaily.* May 5, 2008. Available at: http://www.sciencedaily.com/releases/2008/05 /080504095641.htm. Accessed August 23, 2010.

9. Bio-Medicine. Evidence links protein damage to neurodegenerative diseases like Parkinson's and Alzheimer's. *Bio-Medicine.* November 21, 2000. Available at: http://www.bio-medicine.org/medicine-news/Evidence-Links-Protein-Damage-to-Neurodegenerative-diseases-like-Parkinsons-and-Alzheimers-69-1. Accessed August 23, 2010.

10. Starkman JM. Anesthesia in LBD. *AllExperts.com.* June 6, 2009. Available at: http://en.allexperts.com/q/Anesthesiology-962/2009/6/Anesthesia-LBD.htm. Accessed August 23, 2010.

Chapter 9

1. Whitworth H. LBD travelers extraordinaire. *Lewy Body Digest.* Summer 2007:8. Available at: http://www.lbda.org/category/3477/the-lbda-newsletter.htm. Accessed August 23, 2010.

2. Roehrs T, Roth T. Sleep, sleepiness, and alcohol use. *Alcohol Res Health.* 2001;25(2):101–109. Available at: http://pubs.niaaa.nih.gov/publications/arh25-2/101-109.pdf. Accessed August 23, 2010.

3. Woods DL, Craven RF, Whitney J. The effect of therapeutic touch on behavioral symptoms of persons with dementia [abstract]. *Altern Ther Health Med.* 2005;11(1):66–74. Available at: http://www.ncbi.nlm.nih.gov/pubmed/15712768. Accessed August 23, 2010.

4. Gallaher M. News from the palliative care team. *Beatitudes Campus.* December 2008/January 2009. Available at: http://beatitudescampus.org/content/pub_pcad/PCAD-Issue_2-Dec-Jan-2009.pdf. Accessed August 23, 2010.

5. Selak I. Behavioral issues. *Lewy Body Dementia Association Forum Index.* Available at: http://community.lbda.org/forum. Accessed August 23, 2010.

6. Ferman TJ, Smith GE, Melom B. Understanding behavioral changes in dementia. Lewy Body Dementia Association Web site. 2005. Available at: http://www.lbda.org/index.cfm?fuseaction=docs.download&category_ID=4117&download=1785. Accessed August 23, 2010.

7. Family Care Alliance, Logan B, reviewer. Caregiver's guide to understanding dementia behaviors. Family Caregiver Alliance Web site. 2004. Available at: http://www.caregiver.org/caregiver/jsp/content_node.jsp?nodeid=391. Accessed August 23, 2010.

Chapter 10

1. Anonymous. A patient's point of view. *CARE.* Available at: http://www.pdcaregiver.org/LewyPatient.html. Accessed August 23, 2010.

2. Mayo Clinic staff. Lewy body dementia: preparing for your appointment. *Mayo Clinic.* Available at: http://mayoclinic.com/health/lewy-body-dementia/DS00795/DSECTION=6. Accessed August 23, 2010.

3. Queensland Health Dietitians. Thickened fluids. Queensland government Web site. 2007. Available at: http://www.health.qld.gov.au/nutrition/resources/txt_mod_tf.pdf. Accessed August 23, 2010.

4. Dorner B. It's tough to swallow: a practical approach to nutritional care of dysphagia. National Association Director of Nursing Administrator Long-Term Care Web site. June 15, 2005. Available at: http://stage.nadona.org /media_archive/media/media-72.pdf. Accessed August 23, 2010.

5. Marks J. Constipation. MedicineNet.com. Available at: http://www .medicinenet.com/constipation/article.htm. Accessed August 23, 2010.

6. Riddle R.Constipation: tips from Bay Area support group. *The Lewy Body Dementia Association Forum on Fractical Caregiving Tips.* 2006. Available at: http://community.lbda.org/forum/index.php. Accessed August 23, 2010.

7. Hain TC. Orthostatic hypotension. *Dizziness and Balance.* November 2009. Available at: http://www.dizziness-and-balance.com/disorders /medical/orthostatic.html. Accessed August 23, 2010.

8. Singer W, Sandroni P, Opfer-Gehrking TL, et al. Pyridostigmine treatment trial in neurogenic orthostatic hypotension [abstract]. *Arch Neurol.* April 2006;63(4):513–518. Available at: http://www.ncbi.nlm.nih.gov/pubmed /16476804. Accessed August 23, 2010.

9. Stewart JT. Defining diffuse Lewy body disease: tetrad of symptoms distinguishes illness from other dementias. *Postgrad Med* [serial online]. 2003;113(5):71–75. Available at: http://www.postgradmed.com /index.php?article=1408. Accessed August 23, 2010.

10. Low P. Autonomic nervous system disorders: introduction. *The Merck Manuals Online Medical Library.* 2006. Available at: http://www.merck .com/mmhe/sec06/ch098666/ch098666a.html. Accessed August 23, 2010.

11. Merck Manual. Intimacy and dementia. *The Merck Manual of Health and Aging.* Available at: http://www.merck.com/pubs/mmanual_ha/sec4/ch63 /ch63e.html. Accessed August 23, 2010.

Chapter 11

1. Keren R. Diagnosis and management of dementia with Lewy bodies. *The Canadian Alzheimer's Disease Review.* 2005. Available at: http://www.stacommunications.com/customcomm/Back-issue_pages/AD _Review/adPDFs/2005/june2005e/04.pdf. Accessed August 23, 2010.

2. Walsh N. Growing evidence: cranberry juice tied to lower UTI risk. *BNET.* July 15, 2003. Available at: http://findarticles.com/p/articles/mi_m0CYD /is_14_38/ai_107139817. Accessed August 23, 2010.

Chapter 12

1. ElderCare Neighborhood Network. *ElderCare Online.* Available at: http://www.ec-online.net/Community/Neighborhood/neighborhood.html. Accessed August 23, 2010.

2. Eldercare Online. Available at: http://www.ec-online.net/index.htm. Accessed August 23, 2010.

3. Family Caregiver Alliance. Available at: http://www.caregiver.org/caregiver /jsp/home.jsp. Accessed August 23, 2010.

4. National Association of Area Agencies on Aging. Available at: http://www.n4a.org/about-n4a. Accessed August 23, 2010.

5. Full Circle of Care. Available at: http://www.fullcirclecare.org/index.shtml. Accessed August 23, 2010.

6. US Department of Human Services: Medicare Web site. Available at: http://www.medicare.gov/default.asp. Accessed August 23, 2010.

7. Colorado Foundation for Medical Care. Choosing a home health care agency. Colorado Foundation for Medical Care Web site. Available at: http://www.cfmc.org/consumers/consumers_hh.htm. Accessed August 23, 2010.

8. Assisted Senior Living. Alzheimer's disease centers/dementia caregivers. *Assisted Senior Living.* 2009. Available at: http://www.assistedsenior living.net/ba/alzheimers-disease-dementia-care. Accessed August 23, 2010.

9. National Long-Term Ombudsman Resource Center. Locate an ombudsman, state agencies, and citizen advocacy groups. National Long-Term Ombudsman Resource Center Web site. Available at: http://www .ltcombudsman.org/ombudsman. Accessed August 23, 2010.

10. O'Brien S. How to find the right nursing home. *About.com: Senior Living.* Available at: http://seniorliving.about.com/od/housingoptions /ss/findnursinghome.htm. Accessed August 23, 2010.

Chapter 13

1. Weiner M. Legal and ethical issues for patients with dementia and their families. *Geriatric Times.* January/February 2004. Available at: http://www.cmellc.com/geriatrictimes/g040218.html. Accessed August 23, 2010.

2. LBDA. Brain autopsies and brain donations. Lewy Body Dementia Association Web site. May 1, 2008. Available at: http://www.lbda.org/feature/1949 /brain-autopsies-and-brain-donations.htm. Accessed August 23, 2010.

3. Alzheimer's Association. Social Security Administration for adding early-onset Alzheimer's to its compassionate allowances initiative—Alzheimer's Association statement. *Medical News Today*. Available at: http://www .medicalnewstoday.com/articles/178935.php. Accessed August 23, 2010.

4. Day T. About long term care for veterans. National Care Planning Council Web site. Available at: http://www.longtermcarelink.net/eldercare_veterans _long_term_care.htm. Accessed August 23, 2010.

5. eHow. How to donate your body to science. *eHow*. Available at: http://www.ehow.com/how_110893_donate-body-science.html. Accessed August 23, 2010.

Chapter 14

1. Gordon M. Lewy body disease: end stage. *AllExperts*. April 22, 2007. Available at: http://en.allexperts.com/q/Alzheimer-s-Disease-1005/2008 /4/Lewy-body-disease-end.htm. Accessed August 23, 2010.

2. Medline Plus. Hospice care. *MedlinePlus*. Available at: http://www.nlm .nih.gov/medlineplus/hospicecare.html. Accessed August 23, 2010.

3. Morrison LJ, Liao S. #174: dementia medications in palliative care. Medical College of Wisconsin Web site. Available at: http://www.mcw .edu/fastFact/ff_174.htm. Accessed August 23, 2010.

4. Legacy Home Health Care. Physician's guide to hospice. Legacy Home Health Care & Hospice Web site. Available at: http://www.legacyhome care.com/hospice-physicians-guide. Accessed August 23, 2010.

Chapter 15

1. The White House Conference on Aging. Care for the family caregiver: a place to start. Hip Health Plan of New York, National Alliance for Caregiving Web site. December 2005. Available at: http://www.caregiving .org/pubs/brochures/CFC.pdf. Accessed August 23, 2010.

2. National Alliance for Caregiving. Available at: http://www.caregiving.org. Accessed August 23, 2010.

3. Bear J. What are the stages of grief? *Cancer Survivors On Line*. 2006. Available at: http://www.cancersurvivors.org/Coping/end%20term/stages.htm. Accessed August 23, 2010.

Index

Note: Throughout the Index, the abbreviation LBD is used for Lewy body dementia; AD for Alzheimer's disease; RLS for restless leg syndrome; FDA for Food and Drug Administration; ANS for autonomic nervous system; PDD for Parkinson's disease with dementia; PD for Parkinson's disease; EDS for Excessive daytime sleeping; and LBDA for Lewy Body Dementia Association, Inc. Page numbers followed by *f* indicate figures.